A HALF-CENTURY OF AMERICAN MEDICAL EDUCATION:

1920–1970

A HALF-CENTURY OF AMERICAN MEDICAL EDUCATION:

1920–1970

VERNON W. LIPPARD

Josiah Macy, Jr. Foundation
One Rockefeller Plaza, New York, New York 10020

Contents

Preface

I WAS motivated to write this kind of book by talking with medical students and young faculty members over the lunch table at the Yale School of Medicine and discovering their lack of awareness of events that immediately preceded their entrance into medicine. Even those who were conversant with medical history from Hippocrates to Osler seemed to feel that little had changed over the past fifty years.

The period covered, 1920 to 1970, was not chosen arbitrarily. By 1920 the Flexner Report had had its impact and medical education in the United States was entering a new era. The years around 1970 marked another period of transition. New schools were being opened and older schools were expanding their enrollments. The established pattern of four years of study in college, two years in the basic medical sciences, two years in clinical clerkships, and one year in internship, followed by residency training for specialization, was being abandoned in favor of advanced placement at all levels; early exposure to clinical medicine; more opportunities for elective study; self-instruction with the aid of audiovisual technology and computers; and abbreviation of the total period of training. The introduction of new types of health personnel anticipated a change in the nature of physicians' responsibilities. The economics of medical service were about to be altered, as independent, fee-for-service practice seemed likely to be discarded in favor of a national health program based on prepayment, group practice, and equal access to the system by all income groups.

By chance, this fifty-year period coincided with my own medical career. I entered medical school in 1925 and retired in 1971. The first fourteen of those years were spent as a medical student at Yale and as a resident in pediatrics and a junior faculty member at Cornell and the New York Hospital. Except for a leave for military service in World War II, the next thirty-two were spent in the deans' offices of the College of Physicians and Surgeons at Columbia and the medical schools of Louisiana State University, the University of Virginia, and Yale, with occasional forays into the national and international scenes as an officer of the Association of American Medical Colleges and a member of commissions, conferences, consultant groups, and foundation boards. Consequently the text, although written in the third person, is not entirely impersonal and my prejudices show through. To avoid making it too obviously autobiographical, illustrative personal anecdotes are relegated to footnotes.

This is not a historian's book, replete with charts, graphs, tables, and a complete bibliography, but hopefully it is one that people such as those who inspired me to write it may be interested in reading. The second draft was shorter than the first, and if I had not become impatient the final manuscript would have been even shorter. For those concerned with more detail, the references to monographs and reports of commissions and conferences should be useful because many of them are harder to find in the standard indexes than are articles in the periodical literature, and they include extensive bibliographies.

I am deeply indebted to the Josiah Macy, Jr. Foundation for its support of this publication; to Elizabeth F. Purcell for editing the manuscript; to the Rockefeller Foundation for the opportunity to write part of the first draft while a resident scholar at the Bellagio Study and Conference Center on Lake Como; and to Yale University for providing me with a comfortable study in its Medical Historical Library after my retirement.

Vernon W. Lippard

New Haven
November, 1974

I. Initial Impact of
the Flexner Report

IN 1910, 131 medical schools were in operation in the United States. Five of them had been in existence for more than a hundred years,* but the majority had sprung up in the latter part of the nineteenth century at a time when there was little effort to control quality. While some were at least remotely connected with universities, many were proprietary and operated for profit by their faculties. Admissions standards were low; in fact the only requirement for admission to some of the schools was the ability to pay a tuition fee.

Aware of the deficiencies in the educational programs, leaders in the medical profession had made cautious but largely ineffectual efforts to correct them. The American Medical Association (AMA), founded in 1847, declared among its objectives "cultivating and advancing medical knowledge" and "elevating the standard of medical education." [1] In 1890 representatives of several of the better medical schools met, with similar aims, to form the Association of American Medical Colleges (AAMC).

A few more venerable universities had become uncomfortable about having in their midst professional schools of uncertain quality that offered little more than a series of lectures, repeated annually, and that conferred the degree of doctor of medicine as a reward for attendance. In many instances, however, the connection between the medical schools and their parent universities was so remote that the universities

---

* University of Pennsylvania (1765); Columbia (1767); Harvard (1783); Dartmouth (1797); and University of Maryland (1807). The schools at Pennsylvania, Columbia, and Maryland were founded with different titles, but those in operation a century later were their direct descendants.

had little control over the activities of the schools or failed to accept serious responsibility for their survival. The faculties were composed of practicing physicians who were not dependent on the schools for their livelihoods and whose allegiance was to their professional societies and to the hospitals with which they were associated.

University administrations had made occasional attempts to intervene, with varying degrees of success. As far back as 1827 Yale established Latin and natural philosophy as requirements for admission to medical study, but was forced to retreat when other schools failed to follow and Yale found itself with few medical students.[2]

Under the able leadership of Charles W. Eliot, Harvard was more successful. On assuming the presidency in 1869 Eliot stated that: "The whole system of medical education in this country needs thorough reformation," and proceeded to do something about it locally. In his second annual report he summarized his feelings as follows:

> It seems almost incredible that the grossly inadequate training above described should be the recognized preparation for aspirants to a profession that was once called learned, and which pre-eminently demands a mind well stored and a judgment well trained—a profession in which ignorance is criminality, and skill a benefaction—a profession which penetrates the most sacred retreats of human love, joy and sorrow, and deals daily with the issues of life and death.[3,4]

The reforms instituted during the following few years included establishment of a three-year progressive or graded curriculum (first introduced in 1859 at the Medical Department of Lind University, later to become Northwestern University); extension of courses from four months to a full academic year; reduction in the size of classes; examination of credentials of all applicants; and transfer of financial control to the treasury of the university.

An event of tremendous importance was the establishment of the School of Medicine of the Johns Hopkins University in 1893. With the German universities and their faculties of medicine as a model, and under the inspiring leadership of William Henry Welch, the school introduced methods of instruction and faculty organization that were to be followed by most of the surviving schools over the next thirty years. Teaching and research laboratories became the centers of activity for the basic medical sciences; a university hospital was established and well-organized clinical clerkships were introduced; a substantial nucleus of full-time faculty members, both preclinical and clinical, was appointed; a bachelor's degree was required for admission; and the course of study was extended over four academic years.[5]

Despite a growing dissatisfaction with the current status of medical education, the drastic measures that were needed to change it required the force of a strong national organization. Such an organization had not existed prior to 1901 when the AMA was reorganized in a manner that brought the state medical societies into an organic union as constituent units. One of the first activities of the unified and more influential association was an inquiry into the standards of the medical schools, which revealed the need for a more comprehensive investigation and led to the establishment of the AMA's Council on Medical Education.

It soon became apparent that resentment of the council's criticism of low-grade schools in which influential physicians had stakes would make an impartial survey by the council politically difficult. The Carnegie Foundation for the Advancement of Teaching was invited to take the leadership, with the understanding that the council would be mentioned in the report of the survey only as a source of information.

Abraham Flexner was commissioned in 1908 to make the study and, in company with N. P. Colwell, then secretary of the council, he visited every school in the United States and Canada during the following two years. His report, *Medical Education in the United States and Canada,*[6] published in 1910, was distributed widely and aroused the public to recognition of the fact that the level of medical education in North America was far below that in Europe. The lack of standards, the meager resources, and the incompetent faculties found in many of the schools could no longer be tolerated.

The immediate impact of the report was a remarkable improvement in the standards of medical education. During the next ten years, forty-six of the 131 schools then in existence closed their doors or were absorbed by stronger institutions. Others were strengthened by merger, by university affiliation, and by the infusion of support by private foundations and state governments.

These changes did not take place without a certain amount of pressure. While public opinion and the conscience of the profession undoubtedly played significant roles, the annual publication of a classified list by the council, and the adoption of rules or the passage of state legislation excluding from examinations for licensure the graduates of unapproved schools, put teeth into what might otherwise have been merely pious recommendations.

Within the next few years certain principles were generally accepted, although not immediately adopted, by all schools. To paraphrase H. G. Weiskotten et al.,[7] the foremost were:

1. Preparation for admission to medical school must include enrollment in a college for at least two years, and satisfactory completion of courses in biology, chemistry, and physics.

2. The basic medical sciences must be taught by experienced teachers, trained in their respective subjects, rather than by practicing physicians. The teachers should be scientists who would be prepared to devote their entire time to teaching, investigation, and administration of their departments.

3. Medicine must be learned from observation of the sick and not from books and lectures alone. Adequate clinical facilities must be freely at the disposal of the schools so that they would not be constrained to make faculty appointments merely for the purpose of gaining access to hospital wards.

4. Medical schools should be integrated with the rest of the system of higher education, and should be parts of, or at least affiliated with, universities. As a corollary to this principle it was understood that members of the faculties would have no proprietary interests.

5. Endowment in or support from other sources was considered essential, and schools must not remain dependent on student fees for their financial support.

When the Flexner Report was published, only sixteen schools required two years of college study for admission; about fifty others required only a high school diploma "or its equivalent." The "equivalent" was interpreted broadly, and in actual practice half the students entering many schools had no educational credentials. A by-product of this laissez-faire admissions policy was high attrition, and, in those schools that demanded some degree of achievement, failures during the first year often ran as high as 50 percent. A sharp decrease in failures was observed once the college requirement was established.

The concept of instruction in the basic sciences by scientists rather than by medical practitioners had to be introduced more slowly as trained personnel were not available in sufficient numbers. By 1920, however, most posts in the basic science departments were filled by chemists and biologists, transformed by their special interests into biochemists, anatomists, and physiologists, and by physicians willing to forego practice and be trained on the job. Since the limited salary budgets of the schools were used for faculty members in the foregoing categories, full-time members of clinical departments were scarce.*

Insistence that medical students have access to patients in hospital wards and dispensaries may seem strange today, particularly in view of the inheritance of the British system of medical education which was based in the London hospitals. It must be kept in mind, however, that the poorer schools consisted of little more than lecture halls, and that with rare exceptions the privilege of demonstrating patients was limited to those physicians who, independent of their academic connections, also had control of hospital services.

Institutional affiliations between medical schools and hospi-

---

* The annual budget for the School of Medicine at Yale in 1910–11 was $43,311.

tals were slow in developing.[8] There were similar loose affiliations between medical schools and universities, and many of those in operation before 1910 had none. This situation was corrected, formally if not in practice, and ten years later the majority of the surviving schools had at least nominal university connections.

Most of the surviving schools also found it possible to conform to the rule that they should not be operated on income from tuition fees alone. By 1920 the blatant offenders had closed shop, and state legislators and universities began to recognize medical education as worthy of support. The General Education Board had been established in 1903, and the example it set in providing endowment funds to a selected group of university-affiliated medical schools cannot be overestimated. The board set a standard for stable operation and must have had considerable influence in inducing other private donors to do likewise and in encouraging state legislatures to provide support on an annual basis.

The results of these reforms were not at all favorable. The goal was an elevation of standards, and it was attained gradually. Little attention was paid, however, to quantity in the production of physicians. The system in operation before the Flexner Report at least had the virtue of turning out physicians in numbers sufficient to meet the demands of a rapidly growing and geographically expanding population. Although most of them were general practitioners, who by modern standards were poorly educated and lacking in scientific background, they were available to the inhabitants of the ghettos, the crossroads, and the prairies.

In 1910, 4,400 physicians were graduated in the United States; with the reduction in the number of schools and the application of more strict admissions requirements, by 1920 the number had dropped to 3,047. Half a century passed before the seriousness of this situation was generally recognized and a concerted effort made to correct it.

In summary, the year 1920 marked the beginning of a new era in medical education. Most of the very poor schools had closed and the few remaining were on their way out. Those that survived were ready to start off on a new track.[9]

NOTES

1. M. Fishbein, *A History of the American Medical Association: 1847–1947* (Philadelphia: Saunders, 1947).

2. W. J. Bell, "The Medical Institution of Yale College, 1810–1885," *Yale Journal of Biology and Medicine* 33 (1960): 169.

3. C. W. Eliot, *Annual Reports of the President of Harvard College,* 1869–70, 1870–71.

4. John Z. Bowers, "The Influence of Charles W. Eliot on Medical Education," *The Pharos* 35 (1972): 156.

5. A. M. Chesney, *The Johns Hopkins Hospital and the Johns Hopkins School of Medicine* (Baltimore: Johns Hopkins Press, 1943).

6. A. Flexner, *Medical Education in the United States and Canada* (Carnegie Foundation for the Advancement of Teaching, Bulletin no. 4, 1910).

7. H. G. Weiskotten et al., *Medical Education in the United States: 1934–1939* (Chicago: American Medical Association, 1940).

8. The first university hospital planned and constructed as a teaching facility was opened at the University of Pennsylvania in 1774. See: G. W. Corner, *Two Centuries of Medicine* (Philadelphia: Lippincott, 1965).

9. Far more detailed accounts of American medical education prior to 1920 are available. Among the more comprehensive are: R. H. Shryock, *Medicine and Society in America, 1660–1860* (Ithaca: Cornell University Press, 1962); W. F. Norwood, *Medical Education in the United States before the Civil War* (Philadelphia: University of Pennsylvania Press, 1944); F. R. Packard, *History of Medicine in the United States* (New York: Hoeber, 1931); W. H. Welch, "Medical Education in the United States," *Harvey Lecture* 11 (1916): 366; and C. D. O'Malley, *The History of Medical Education* (Berkeley: University of California Press, 1970).

II. Curriculum

B Y 1920 the course of study in the better medical schools was moving toward a pattern that was to prevail over the next fifty years. Those that could not measure up to the accepted standards, in terms of facilities, faculties, and teaching programs, were destined to close.

A minimum requirement of two years of study in a liberal arts college prior to admission was generally accepted, although most schools required three years, and a few a bachelor's degree. A basic knowledge of biology, general and organic chemistry, and physics was considered essential.

The graded curriculum had replaced the lectures, repeated annually, that had been the common practice only a few years earlier. The program covered four academic years, and students were advanced on successful completion of rigid examinations. Those who failed individual courses were allowed to be reexamined or to repeat the year, but those who failed in courses that approximated half the required hours were dismissed. The first year was a grueling experience for students who did not possess retentive memories. The study of gross anatomy was a major hurdle, and many young people who showed promise of becoming good physicians fell by the wayside because of their inability to describe the articular facets of the femur or the origin and insertion of the gastrocnemius muscle.

The first year was devoted to study of gross and microscopic anatomy, biochemistry, and physiology. Approximately half the scheduled hours were spent in anatomy laboratories, principally dissecting rooms, where each student teased out the fascia and removed the fat to expose and recognize every organ, nerve, muscle, bone, and blood vessel in the human body and associate it with the appropriate Latin nomenclature.

As each structure was exposed, the student referred to his worn and grease-spotted volume of Gray's *Anatomy,* then in its twentieth American edition, which rested on a stand at the head of the table, and dreamed of the day he would possess a stethoscope and examine a live patient.

Biochemistry, in some schools called "physiological chemistry," was a recent offshoot of physiology and was becoming recognized as the most important foundation for understanding scientific medicine. It dealt largely with nutrition and intermediary metabolism on what fifty years later would be considered a superficial level. Lectures were supplemented by laboratory exercises that were similar to those the students had experienced in college. Each so-called experiment was described step by step in a laboratory manual, and success was determined by ability to crystallize out a component of the blood or urine, or measure its concentration by the colorimetric or gravimetric methods. In retrospect one wonders how much these exercises contributed to an understanding of physiological processes, but they were prescribed religiously in the curriculum of every school.

The remaining quarter of the first year was devoted to the study of physiology, which for most students was the most exciting experience. Although the laboratory manuals dictated the experiments and allowed for no ingenuity, the fact remained that one was dealing with living organisms ranging from frogs to one's fellow students. The major apparatus was the kymograph, a machine operated by clockworks that rotated a cylinder or drum covered with smoked paper. Muscle contractions and pressure changes caused a lever to fluctuate and scratch the surface of the rotating drum. Although much time was spent in smoking the paper and adjusting the lever, operating on anesthetized animals and observing physiological responses were absorbing experiences.

The schedule for the second year usually included courses in pathology, bacteriology, pharmacology, and an introduction to clinical medicine. In pathology, the study of disease, the student at last began to feel like a doctor, as he examined diseased organs and tissues, grossly and microscopically, and attended autopsies on patients who had died in the hospital.

The course in bacteriology was clinically oriented. The morphological and cultural characteristics of pathogenic bacteria and other microorganisms were studied in the lecture hall and laboratory, and students learned to perform serological examinations such as the Wassermann and Widal reactions.

In most schools there was also a course known as "laboratory medicine" or "clinical pathology" in which the students learned diagnostic procedures such as blood counts, urinalyses, liver function tests, and examination of stools for parasites. As a result, the young physician in the 1920s came far closer to being able to perform the standard diagnostic tests then in common use than his counterpart fifty years later.

Pharmacology, as it was taught at that time, was a strange mixture of prescription writing and demonstrations or laboratory exercises in which the effects of drugs on laboratory animals were observed. In some schools time was wasted in compounding pills and ointments, even though the day when physicians dispensed medicines in their offices had passed.

Toward the end of the second year a course in physical diagnosis, which included history taking, introduced the student to clinical medicine. Equipped with a stethoscope and a clean white coat he ventured timorously onto the open wards, listened intently for bronchial breathing, crepitant rales, or premature systoles, and gradually overcame a terrible sense of insecurity. At last he was being rewarded for the hours of drudgery in the anatomy laboratory.

Most physicians raised in the system that prevailed from the 1920s through the 1960s look back on the next two years, the third and fourth years in medical school, as the period in their lives when they worked the longest hours, studied the hardest, learned the most, and were the most exhilarated. Although American medical schools had adopted the German system of education in the basic medical sciences, they had fortunately been guided by the British system in developing the program for the two clinical years. The clinical clerkship program, in which the student rotates through a series of clinical services and takes part in the care of patients under close supervision, has stood the test of time and is now considered as satisfactory an educational experience as it was fifty years ago.

One of the virtues of this method of education is that it is never behind the times. The patients that one sees in the outpatient clinics and hospital wards are suffering from diseases that are prevalent today, and the diagnostic and therapeutic methods in use are the most advanced—they are not reflections of worn-out textbooks or last year's lecture notes. The syllabus, if there were one, would change from year to year.

Over the period under consideration in this book the time devoted to the study of various diseases changed tremendously. In the 1920s, patients suffering from infectious diseases occupied a large percentage of the hospital beds. Mortality from some types of pneumonia was high, and bacteriological diagnosis and use of the appropriate antiserum, if available, were of paramount importance. The incidence of tuberculosis remained high, and heroic measures such as collapse of the infected lung by increasing pressure in the pleural space by air injection, or removal of ribs, were in common use. Children with diphtheria, scarlet fever, and congenital syphilis required a great deal of attention. Infantile diarrhea and related marasmus were major problems on the infants' wards. With the introduction of antibiotics, improved sanitation, and other preventive measures the incidence of these diseases decreased, as did the time in the curriculum devoted to them—not by any formal procedure but because what was taught on the wards and in the outpatient clinics was governed by the disorders of the patients who were seen there.

The ability to perform a normal delivery was considered, in the 1920s, one of the essential skills of every physician, and a requirement that a certain number of deliveries had been performed was stated in the regulations governing licensure in many states. Most teaching hospitals had large obstetrical services for charity patients where students were allowed to exercise their talents. Deliveries in the home were still common, and performance of deliveries in "the district" not only provided the students with exciting and rewarding experiences they were delighted to relate, but gave them an exposure to ethnic, cultural, and environmental situations that was never equalled in the more contrived programs in comprehensive medicine developed later.

Changes in the content of clinical courses were determined by scientific advances and by the distribution of illnesses in the hospital populations. With advances in biochemical knowledge, metabolism and endocrinology played more important roles in internal medicine. Surgeons became more aware of the physiological changes that resulted from surgical trauma and anesthesia and gave more attention to pre- and postoperative care. In pediatrics there was increased emphasis on physical, mental, and social growth and development, and on neonatalogy and genetics. Instruction in obstetrics was no longer confined to the detection of pregnancy and the mechanisms of labor, but gave new emphasis to reproductive biology, including contraception and the management of sterility.

In the basic sciences, scientific advances rather than changes in methods of instruction determined the emphasis given to courses and topics. Introduction of the electron microscope made possible the study of the morphology of subcellular elements and broadened the scope of courses in microscopic anatomy. Instruction in biochemistry became more concerned with enzyme systems and biochemical genetics. Physiologists became more interested in the study of fundamental processes, such as membrane permeability and nerve conduction, than in organ function. Pharmacologists became more biochemically oriented and, until the introduction of a new breed of clinical pharmacologists who combined interest in basic pharmacology and clinical medicine, more divorced from therapeutics. Bacteriology departments were appropriately redesignated departments of microbiology, ceased to be concerned with identification of bacteria, and dealt more extensively with viruses and other microorganisms as well as microbial genetics.

The summation of all these developments in the fields of interest of basic science faculties resulted not only in a change in the scope of material covered in their courses but, more important, in their divorce from clinical medicine. The basic scientist with a Ph.D. and narrow interests was seldom capable of interpreting the relationship of the basic sciences to human biology and disease. Fortunately, many young physicians who, during the years after World War II, were trained both as clinicians and as scientists in limited fields were able to assume this responsibility.

Schedule Adjustments

In 1920 the course of study was based on the assumption that after graduation and a year or two of internship the young physician would be prepared to enter general practice and deal with almost any problem presented, including most major surgery. Consequently, nothing could be left out and the volume of material covered became greater and greater and the course more and more superficial. This led to a good deal of unrest on the part of faculty members who felt that important areas of their specialization were not being adequately covered. Furthermore, students became aware of the trend toward specialization and were less willing to postpone some degree of concentration until the postgraduate years.

Something had to give, and the adjustment was brought about in two ways: by decreasing the hours devoted to some subjects, and increasing the length of the course by extending the academic year. The subject that suffered the greatest loss of hours was gross anatomy, which at the beginning of this period was assigned four hundred to six hundred hours, and at the end approximately two hundred. While in the 1920s the program leading to the medical degree occupied four academic years, each of approximately thirty-two weeks, by the end of the 1960s the average year was nearer thirty-six weeks and many schools required the student to be in residence during most of one or two summers.

These adjustments opened the way to the introduction of more elective courses and opportunities for research. The extent of these innovations, however, differed widely among the schools. The more conservative faculties stuck to rigid programs, in which every minute was accounted for, backed up by frequent examinations; the more liberal faculties decreased the number of classroom and required laboratory hours. It was not until the end of the era under consideration that elective programs became more or less structured. Time had to be found for subjects that had previously been neglected: principally preventive medicine, the behavioral sciences, and psychiatry.

INTRODUCTION OF NEW DISCIPLINES

Courses in hygiene, later labeled public health or preventive medicine, were introduced early in the twentieth century and gradually found their way into most medical curricula. It cannot be said, however, that they gained universal popularity. While students readily grasped the importance of immunization, pre- and postpartum examinations, control of venereal disease, and improved sanitation, visits to sewage disposal plants and city health departments left them cold and were eventually abandoned. Physicians were sympathetic to public health measures and generally cooperative in adopting them when they involved the care of individual patients, but even after the sciences of biometry and epidemiology had become well developed it was difficult to arouse much excitement about health measures for large population groups.

Toward the end of the period one aspect of the rather ill-defined discipline sometimes designated "social" or "community" medicine, aroused the interest of many socially conscious students. Better distribution of health services, with emphasis on greater accessibility to medical care by the disadvantaged, became a political issue and a rallying point for the liberals.

In the early years of the twentieth century instruction in psychiatry was confined to a series of lectures supplemented by demonstration of patients, usually with well-established syndromes, at a mental hospital. There was little in this experience to stimulate the student to explore the field more deeply, and it is not surprising that the study of mental diseases occupied an isolated position.

The most significant contributions of science to medicine depended on the impact of physics and chemistry on biology and the introduction of quantitative biological methods. While this concept fostered the approach that man, an isolated biological unit, could be understood by investigation of his genetic biological endowment alone, it failed to take into account the influence of interpersonal and cultural factors on human personality development and physiological functions. This situation prevailed through World War II, and although there was some awakening of interest in psychiatry during the war it was not until later that departments on a par with those of medicine and surgery, or even pediatrics and obstetrics, were established. The change in attitude of medical faculties probably would have occurred anyway, but it was hastened by the observation that the average armed forces medical officer found himself devoting a good share of his time to dealing with neuroses and psychosomatic disorders generated by the stresses of military life.

The introduction of full-time faculty members and research programs in psychiatry was reflected in a dramatic change in the curriculum, interest in which was stimulated, or at least crystallized, by the 1951 Conference on Psychiatric Education, held at Cornell University.[1] Thereafter, most schools introduced the behavioral sciences in the first year with a course in personality development, provided some background in psychotherapy in the second year, and offered clinical clerkships in psychiatric divisions of general hospitals or in mental hospitals in the third and fourth years.

Formal courses in the history of medicine were also introduced during this period. When H. E. Sigerist made a survey in 1939, medical history had gained departmental status in only one school—Johns Hopkins; there were few other professional historians in the field.[2] Elsewhere, occasional lectures by faculty members in a variety of departments represented the total offering. Thirty years later, sixteen schools had full-time professors, and several of them had graduate programs leading to advanced degrees.[3] This somewhat optimistic appraisal of progress in the field was tempered by the observation that medical history was a required course in only fourteen of the schools, and elective in twenty-five others.

Not only the subject matter but the methods of instruction changed. Although lectures prevailed, and even textbook assignments and recitations were not uncommon at the beginning of this era, by the end of it the former had diminished in frequency and importance and the latter had been abandoned entirely. When the study of medicine was at the college level it was not surprising that college methods of instruction would be used; when it shifted to the graduate level, however, most schools failed to make the appropriate adjustments.

The Yale Program

The first radical departure from traditional methods was made at Yale, where in 1925 what became known at the "Yale System" was introduced under the dynamic leadership of Milton C. Winternitz.[4] This plan had four main characteristics: lack of fixed course requirements; emphasis on elective courses; absence of required examinations and grades in individual courses; and a required dissertation based on original investigation. Students were encouraged to advance at their own pace, and those who had previous experience in the basic medical sciences could fit into the program without repeating courses. There were fewer than the usual scheduled hours in the curriculum, and more elective options permitted the student to pursue his special interests in depth. Comprehensive examinations were offered at the end of the preclinical and clinical periods. To meet the requirements for the dissertation, the student was expected, with guidance, to explore the literature in a chosen field; formulate a hypothesis; work out a method of approach; carry out the necessary experiments; and write an acceptable report.

The basic philosophy of this program was summarized in a faculty report written several years after its inauguration:

Fundamental to this program is the concept that the student is a mature individual, is strongly motivated to learn and requires guidance and stimulation rather than compulsion or competition for relative standing in his group. Equally basic is the concept that if the student is given unusual privileges, he must assume more than the usual responsibility for his education.[5]

Although no other school adopted a similar program immediately, its influence was far-reaching. Over the years the curricula of all schools became more flexible, lectures and examinations were deemphasized, and opportunities for elective study and research expanded.

THE WESTERN RESERVE PROGRAM

The equilibrium—or complacency—of the faculties was seriously disturbed by the outbreak of World War II. Large numbers of physicians entered the military services; medical scientists and educators took part in war-associated activities; the curriculum was accelerated and the internship period shortened; and brilliant scientific advances were made in all fields of medicine. A new mass of accumulated medical knowledge was added to the already overloaded medical curriculum, and faculty and students were faced with an insuperable task. The time was ripe for a reconsideration of the established curriculum.

Among the several curricular innovations of the postwar period, the program that was most carefully developed, and the one that had the greatest impact, was introduced at Western Reserve University in 1952.* Under the leadership of Joseph J. Wearn and T. Hale Ham, a curriculum was developed that abandoned all thought of total coverage. Emphasis was placed on basic concepts; the mechanisms of disease; continuing self-education; the development of a scientific critique; the cultivation of skills; and the inculcation of ideals. Although the departmental structure of the school

* In 1967 Western Reserve University merged with the Case Institute of Technology to become Case Western Reserve University.

remained unchanged for administrative purposes, teaching by discipline was discontinued and the program was planned by interdisciplinary subject committees.

The four-year curriculum was divided into three phases: the first, lasting one year, was concerned with normal structure, function, growth, and development; the second, lasting one-and-one-half years, was concerned with alterations of normal structure, function, and development, and the study of disease; the third, also lasting one-and-one-half years, was devoted to the clinical application of the knowledge previously acquired.

The students' objection to the standard curriculum of the time, two years of preclinical and two of clinical studies, was that preclinical studies were merely intellectual hurdles that had to be overcome in order to enter their chosen field of clinical medicine. Arrangement of the first two phases of the program by systems, such as the cardiovascular system and the nervous system, and by etiology, such as infectious diseases, was thought to provide an integrated framework of knowledge that the physician would use throughout his career. Early contact with patients made the study of the basic sciences more meaningful.

Integration of instruction by systems, which characterized the first two phases, was less practical in the third phase. The sixteen calendar months assigned to this phase was divided into eight months of compulsory clerkships in the wards and outpatient services, six of electives, and two of vacation. Throughout this period emphasis was placed on continuity of relationships among the student and his group of colleagues. Many other interesting aspects of this program that cannot be covered in this brief review are described elsewhere.[6]

Although the Western Reserve system was not adopted in toto by any other medical school it had an enormous influence on the attitudes of other faculties, and particularly on the planning of curricula for new schools. Several settled on a compromise that provided for traditional disciplinary instruction in the basic medical sciences during the first year or year-and-a-half, followed by an integrated interdisciplinary course arranged by systems.[7]

A by-product of this experiment was the introduction of multidisciplinary laboratories for instruction in the basic sciences. Heretofore all schools had separate student laboratories for each department, which represented an extravagant use of space because most of them were vacant at least half the year. Each student or group of students had a bench and locker in each of the several laboratories and the size of classes was limited accordingly. The multidisciplinary laboratories provided facilities for chemical, physiological, and microscopic experiments and study, so that each student had a base for all of his laboratory work. The laboratories were arranged in units that accommodated approximately sixteen students, and were serviced from a central supply room. This design, first developed at Western Reserve, was refined when the Stanford University School of Medicine consolidated its activities and erected a new physical plant on the Palo Alto campus. With various modifications, it was used in the construction of almost all of the new schools that were opened during the following twenty years.

Another consequence of the Western Reserve program was the interest it stimulated in the evaluation of medical curricula and teaching methods. Medical educators, like those in other graduate and professional schools, had not been interested in appraising the results of educational experiments and conducting controlled experiments in pedagogy. From time to time educational psychologists had studied the admissions process and individual courses, but efforts to evaluate entire curricula were almost unknown. In 1958 Western Reserve organized a Division of Research in Medical Education, with studies of that type as its major objective. Also active in introducing educational research were the medical schools of the universities of Buffalo, Illinois, and Southern California. By 1970 similar units were in operation at approximately half the schools listed in the AAMC Directory. The studies and provocative reports of George E. Miller and his associates in the Division of Research in Medical Education of the University of Illinois played a major role in stimulating interest in this field.[8]

Comprehensive Medicine

In the 1950s the faculties of several schools realized with concern that because they had become so involved in teaching the vast body of empirical knowledge, little attention was being given to its effective application. A conscious effort appeared to be indicated to interest the student in obtaining a broad understanding of the patient, including the pertinent psychological, social, and cultural factors. This rather vague concept was designated as "comprehensive medicine." General medical clinics were established, to which both adult and pediatric patients were admitted, and students were given the opportunity to follow their patients over periods of several months. Consultations with specialists and social workers were made readily available. While the treatment of biological problems was carried out in the usual manner, greater emphasis was placed on emotional and environmental factors that influenced the patient's reaction to his illness. The conduct of these clinics and their impact on the patient, the student, and the quality of medical service were studied by sociologists and psychologists at Cornell, Colorado, Pennsylvania, and Western Reserve universities.[9-11] As this concept was introduced at about the same time as improved instruction in psychiatry and social medicine was being stressed, it is difficult to determine which had the greater influence on the attitudes of the students.

To many, the whole movement seemed rather contrived: they questioned, with considerable justification, whether students acquire compassion, understanding, and social conscience by exposure to comprehensive clinics, home care programs, apprenticeships with country physicians and general practitioners, or courses in sociology. In his presidential address to the Association of American Physicians in 1955, Robert F. Loeb pleaded "that we maintain the emphasis in undergraduate education on intellectual growth and thereby guard against the subtle encroachments of romanticism." [12]

THE STANFORD PROGRAM

The idea that four academic years was the proper time span for the medical course had become so firmly established that it took a great deal of courage to challenge it. The size of the box had been determined and faculties were expected to fit whatever they chose into it, instead of deciding first on the contents and constructing the box accordingly. In the 1950s this concept began to be questioned. Several schools extended the clinical clerkships into the summers between the second and third or third and fourth years, thereby not only increasing the length of the course but utilizing clinical facilities more efficiently. More radical departures were illustrated in the programs put into operation at Stanford, Johns Hopkins, Northwestern, and Boston universities.

The Stanford plan, inaugurated in 1959, was based on three major concepts: (1) that all education is a continuum; (2) that while the growth of medical science is so great and continues at so rapid a pace that comprehensive coverage cannot be achieved, there is a core of medical knowledge that should be presented to all students; and (3) that the student of medicine has passed beyond that stage of his education where mere acquisition of "facts" can be defended.[13] In designing the new curriculum, many of the policies introduced at Yale thirty-five years earlier were adopted: greater flexibility and opportunity for elective work and original research; and a deemphasis on didactic teaching, examinations, and grades. Instruction in the basic sciences was integrated in a pattern similar to that introduced at Western Reserve a few years before. The unusual feature of the Stanford plan was extension of the period of registration in the medical school from four to five years. The period devoted to preclinical studies was extended from two to three years, but approximately one-third of each of these years could be used for study elsewhere in the university in accordance with the student's interests.

THE JOHNS HOPKINS PROGRAM

The combined college-medical school program at Johns Hopkins, which also went into effect in the fall of 1959, was based on many of the same assumptions.[14] The program incorporated most of the same policies, such as greater flexibility and the merging of instruction in the liberal arts and medical science. It differed sharply from the Stanford plan, however, in that it was designed to decrease, rather than maintain or increase, the period between college entrance and award of the M.D. degree. This decision was based on the conviction that the number of years required for students to reach a productive stage in practice or research had gradually grown to the point where able students were becoming reluctant to enter the field of medicine. The period of postdoctoral training for most graduates was three to five years and, with two years of military services added, the average physician was thirty to thirty-two years of age by the time he could earn a living.

Under the Hopkins plan, students could be admitted to the combined program at the end of their sophomore or junior year in college. The curriculum consisted of five forty-week years. Those admitted without bachelors' degrees were registered in both the college and medical school and enrolled in courses on both campuses during the first year. Those with bachelors' degrees entered directly into the second year of the program and took the courses usually offered in the first year of medical school. Students were then permitted to accelerate their required work in the clinical years, by electing required courses in free quarters and the intervening summer, so that they were ready to enter internships in the fifth year. The M.D. degree was awarded at the end of five years. Thus the student who took full advantage of the opportunity to accelerate could graduate from medical school and complete his internship in seven instead of nine calendar years from the time he entered college.

THE NORTHWESTERN PROGRAM

At Northwestern University a six-year program leading to the M.D. degree was initiated in the fall of 1961 for a group of twenty-five students entering directly from high school.[15] The program was designed for highly talented students who could qualify for advanced college placement on the basis of superior achievement both in high school and in examinations. Approximately one hundred other students were admitted in the usual way after four years of college.

Under the six-year plan, the first two years were spent on the university campus at Evanston. A unique feature of the program during this period was the organization of special courses in the sciences for these students. A combined physics-mathematics course presented key concepts and theories and encouraged the development of intellectual tools as a basis for advanced study in any science. The chemistry course, running throughout the two years, emphasized the more physical approaches and areas basic to the study of biological systems. The biology course in the second year had the advantage of being based on the content of the already completed courses in mathematics, physics, and chemistry. These science courses occupied half the classroom hours, the other half being devoted to English, behavioral sciences, and electives. At the end of the second year, students moved to the medical center campus in Chicago, and over the next four years followed the same curriculum as students admitted after graduating from college.

It was recognized that the success of this experiment would be contingent on careful selection. Apparently the selection process was adequate because it was reported subsequently that these six-year students did as well or better than the average in medical school. To many observers, however, that was not a convincing argument in favor of abbreviating the educational program for all prospective physicians. The maturation that takes place during a longer and broader liberal arts education was held to be necessary, or at least desirable, for most students.

A similar six-year program was announced by Boston University in 1961,[16] with the ultimate intention of admitting essentially the entire class directly from high school. While it was still in operation a decade later, the majority of students entering the medical school in 1971 had had the usual college preparation.

The adoption of the Johns Hopkins, Northwestern, and Boston university programs, which shortened the students' formal education for the M.D. degree, forecast a more widespread movement in that direction over the following ten years. By 1970 approximately a quarter of the schools in the United States had made it possible for a student to elect to graduate from medical school at the end of three rather than four calendar years. This was accomplished by reducing vacation periods rather than by decreasing the actual weeks of instruction, which remained in the neighborhood of one hundred and forty. Many faculties seriously resisted this trend because it diminished opportunities for elective experiences such as research, substitute internships, and intensive study in areas of interest during the summer vacations.

Other Innovations in the 1960s

Dissatisfaction with the traditional curriculum was manifested in other ways during the late 1960s, when there was growing pressure to increase the production of physicians, and when new schools were being opened and existing schools were expanding their enrollments. Society was demanding that medical schools admit a greater number of students from geographic areas, economic backgrounds, and ethnic groups that had previously been inadequately represented. Moreover, students were revolting against the standardized course of study, and wanted education individualized to fit their varying rates of achievement, diverse educational backgrounds, and differing career goals. The fact that the curriculum was over-loaded with factual information—which some had recognized twenty years earlier—was becoming more and more apparent.

In response to these pressures the faculties of one school after another undertook serious analyses of their programs. The first to announce a solution was Duke University, where a drastic change was put into effect in the fall of 1965.[17] The new curriculum consisted of three phases. During Phase I, covering the first academic year, those aspects of the basic medical sciences which it was thought every student should know were presented, with emphasis on principles rather than details. Less time was spent in teaching laboratories, and demonstrations were used more extensively. Phase II, extending through the second academic year, was devoted to clinical clerkships in medicine, surgery, pediatrics, obstetrics and gynecology, and psychiatry. In Phase III, extending through the third and fourth years, each student's course of study was tailored to his interests and capabilities. A program was organized for each individual, in consultation with two advisors.

Within the next five years almost every school in the country adopted a program organized along similar lines.[18,19] The core curriculum in the basic sciences varied from one to two academic years. Instead of the standard six-course program, interdisciplinary instruction was introduced and course titles such as cell biology, growth and development, and neural sciences were substituted. Many schools devoted a portion of the second year to instruction by systems and etiologies. Adoption of a basic or required clerkship extending over one academic year was almost universal. This phase of the curriculum was disturbed the least, and it seems apparent that an apprenticeship in dealing with patients, under close supervision in a university hospital, was considered by most faculties to be essential.

The most extensive and widely adopted change was the introduction of an elective period covering the last year or year-and-a-half. Even the schools that for decades had scheduled almost every minute over the four years in required courses, each followed by an examination, made provision for the pursuit of special interests. The extent to which the elective periods were controlled varied widely at the beginning, from complete freedom of choice to structured "tracks" or "pathways" in broad areas involving clinical work and study of the relevant basic sciences. Although descriptions of these programs invariably stated that the student would explore in depth those aspects of the basic sciences related to his career goals, the opportunities were, by 1970, poorly developed. Many of the more successful elective courses in the basic sciences were offered by members of clinical rather than basic science departments. The success or failure of this curriculum, which at the outset was conceptually so sound, depended upon how efficiently the elective period was utilized.

NOTES

1. J. C. Whitehorn et al., eds., *Psychiatry and Medical Education,* Report of the 1951 Conference on Psychiatric Education (Washington, D.C.: American Psychiatric Association, 1952).

2. H. E. Sigerist, "Medical History in the Medical Schools of the United States," *Bulletin of the History of Medicine* 7 (1939): 627.

3. G. Miller, "The Status of Medical History in the Universities of North America and Europe: I. The Teaching of Medical History in the United States and Canada," *Bulletin of the History of Medicine* 43 (1969): 259.

4. See: R. Hussey, "The Study of Medicine at Yale," *Yale Journal of Biology and Medicine* 1 (1928): 18; and S. C. Harvey, "The Objectives of Medical Education," ibid., 13 (1941): 847; reprinted ibid., 26 (1953): 8.

5. V. W. Lippard, "The Yale Plan of Medical Education after Thirty Years," *Journal of Medical Education* 29 (1954): 17.

6. T. H. Ham, "Medical Education at Western Reserve University: A Progress Report for Sixteen Years, 1946–1962," *New England Journal of Medicine* 267 (1962): 868. (Contains extensive bibliography of earlier reports on this program.)

7. M. L. Karnovsky, "Unified Approach to Basic Medical Sciences at Harvard," *Journal of Medical Education* 30 (1955): 15.

8. G. E. Miller, *Teaching and Learning in Medical School* (Cambridge: Harvard University Press, 1961).

9. F. Kern and K. R. Hammond, "Research in Teaching of Comprehensive Medicine," *Journal of Medical Education* 31 (1956): 535.

10. G. G. Reader, "Some of the Problems and Satisfactions of

Teaching Comprehensive Medicine," *Journal of Medical Education* 31 (1956): 544.

11. R. K. Merton, S. Bloom, and N. Rogoff, "Studies in the Sociology of Medical Education," *Journal of Medical Education* 31 (1956): 552.

12. R. F. Loeb, "Values in Undergraduate Medical Education," *Transactions of Association of American Physicians* 68 (1955): 1.

13. L. M. Stowe, "The Stanford Plan: An Educational Continuum for Medicine," *Journal of Medical Education* 34 (1959): 1059.

14. "A Revised Program of Medical Education at Johns Hopkins," *Journal of Medical Education* 33 (1958): 225. (Reprinted from *The Johns Hopkins Magazine* 8, no. 9 [June 1957].)

15. J. A. D. Cooper and M. Prior, "A New Program in Medical Education at Northwestern University," *Journal of Medical Education* 36 (1961): 80.

16. P. V. Lee, *Medical Schools and the Changing Times: Nine Case Reports on Experiments in Medical Education, 1950–1960* (Evanston: Association of American Medical Colleges, 1962).

17. H. O. Sieker, "A New Curriculum for Medical Education," *Clinical Research* 13 (1965): 3.

18. V. W. Lippard and Elizabeth Purcell, eds., *The Changing Medical Curriculum,* Report of a Macy Conference (New York: Josiah Macy, Jr. Foundation, 1972). (Contains detailed descriptions of typical new curricula in operation in 1970–71.)

19. *AAMC Curriculum Directory: 1972–1973* (Washington, D.C.: Association of American Medical Colleges, 1972). (Contains outlines of curricula of all medical schools in the United States and Canada.)

III. The Medical Student
and His Environment

THE requirement of two or three years of education at the college level prior to admission to medical school had, by 1920, become well established and an increasing number of students were entering with bachelors' degrees. There was less competition for admission than there was to be later, and the selection process was not so well organized. Committees on admissions existed in many schools, at least on paper, but they were not overworked and most of the responsibility for the selection of students rested with the dean or assistant dean. He read application forms, transcripts of college grades, and letters of recommendation, interviewed prospective students, and made the ultimate decision.

The attitude of the average dean may be summarized in the comments of R. C. Lewis, an assistant dean at Columbia, in a discussion of admission practices at the 1930 meeting of the AAMC. He said, in part:

> Scholarship grades mean one thing in one place and another thing at another place. Until the Committee becomes sufficiently familiar with the actual value of a grade of 75 or 80 at a given school, I do not think they are in a position to know whether a man having such a grade at such a school is capable of doing the work in this particular [medical] school. Recommendations come second in deceptiveness, perhaps, to statistics. I should say that nine-tenths of the recommendations that we get in our school are valueless from the point of view of actually rating the applicant as a desirable student. I doubt that we shall ever be willing to give up the personality test by meeting applicants for a personal interview.[1]*

* When I occupied the same position ten years later the system and the policies remained the same.

With the exception of disgruntled relatives of rejected applicants, most people thought this system worked quite well. Medical students were, by and large, clean-cut young fellows who worked hard enough to get by and turned out to be good doctors. There were, however, those who felt that the system should be improved, and the AAMC established the Committee on Scholastic Aptitude Test, with F. A. Moss of George Washington University as its secretary and director of studies. The committee devised what became known as the "Medical Aptitude Test," or the "Moss Test," and reported on a two-year trial at the 1930 AAMC meeting.[2] Dr. Moss pointed out that the test was not intended to measure general intelligence, but rather to predict success in medical studies. Apparently it did just that; there was a fairly good correlation between test scores and success or failure in the preclinical courses of the first two years. The test was administered at colleges across the country, under the direction of the AAMC, and the results reported to the medical schools. It is unfortunate that it became known as an "aptitude" test because it certainly did not measure vocational aptitude.

The test was used as an adjunct to the methods of selection described earlier, but most deans remained skeptical and thought it added little to information available in the college records. Their attitude may be summarized by the comments of another assistant dean, this one from Harvard:

> Just as medical diagnosis is aided by the laboratory, the selection of medical students is improved by using more than one test. But both in medicine and in the admission office tests should take their proper place and no more. The prognosis for both patient and applicant is to be determined clinically and not with an adding machine.[3]

In the meantime, under the sponsorship of the Carnegie Foundation for the Advancement of Teaching, the Graduate Record Examination was inaugurated as an experiment in selecting students for admission to graduate schools. First offered on a national basis in 1943, the examination was promptly accepted as an important credential. It provided scores in mathematics, physics, chemistry, biological science, history and economics, literature, fine arts, and verbal skills. The scores represented the relative standing of the students with respect to their knowledge of these subject areas. Reported in terms of standard scores, a student's aptitude in one subject area could be compared directly with his performance in other areas, as well as with the performances of other individuals or groups of students. An examination of this type had a good deal of appeal to those who were dissatisfied with the Moss Medical Aptitude Test which, after a trial of fifteen years, had been discarded.

The Medical College Admissions Test (MCAT),[4] first administered in 1948, had many of the characteristics of the Graduate Record Examination. It consisted of four sections, each of which was separately timed, scored, and reported: (1) verbal ability; (2) the understanding and interpretation of qualitative material; (3) knowledge and ability to reason in the social sciences; and (4) knowledge of elementary biology, chemistry, and physics, and ability to grasp the fundamental principles of science. The MCAT was developed and administered for the AAMC by the Educational Testing Service, and later by the Psychological Corporation. Within a year or two it was being administered twice yearly at colleges across the country, and was required to be taken by applicants to all medical schools. Numerous studies in later years supported the impression that the MCAT was a useful adjunct to college records, recommendations, and interviews, although no school was willing to depend on it alone.[5] While the MCAT was still in common use twenty years later, its relation to a student's success as a physician, rather than just his ability to do well in medical school, had never been established.

With the introduction of such tests the admissions process became more formal. The demand for admission increased as large numbers of veterans of World War II, aided by the G.I. Bill of Rights, made plans to enter medical schools. Members of admissions committees participated in the interviewing of candidates and had a stronger voice in the decisions.

In the early part of this period, little attention was given to the student's course of study in college provided he met the minimal science requirements. Actually, most students followed what was known as the "premedical course," which usually included general biology, comparative anatomy of vertebrates and invertebrates, embryology, general and organic chemistry, quantitative and qualitative analyses, and physics. Various combinations of these subject areas were required for admission to different medical schools, as was a reading knowledge of French or German.

Prompted by a concern for the admission of students with a broader liberal arts education, the John and Mary R. Markle Foundation sponsored a committee which in 1953 published the report, *Preparation for Medical Education in a Liberal Arts College.*[6] The principal recommendation of this study was to limit the course requirements to biology, general and organic chemistry, and physics, and to eliminate the necessity for the student to take other science courses in order to be eligible for consideration at several schools. A secondary recommendation, and the one of most interest to the committee, was to improve the opportunity of the student who anticipated a career in medicine to obtain a broader background in the humanities and social sciences. It also encouraged the student who made a late, and often more mature, decision to go to medical school, because he could complete the essential science courses in his junior and senior years.

The Student Body

The student of the 1920s and 1930s, having entered medical school at the age of twenty-one or twenty-two, engaged in serious study, usually without interruption and with few distractions, for four successive years. In this respect he differed from his counterpart in England, who began his medical studies earlier, and who could, at the same time, engage in undergraduate organized athletics and social affairs. The American medical student's life also differed from that of his contemporaries in graduate school—candidates for the Ph.D. degree—who progressed with less regularity.

During the first two years, classes began at eight o'clock in the morning and continued until late in the afternoon, five-and-a-half days a week for thirty-two to thirty-six weeks. The total number hours of lectures and laboratory exercises amounted to approximately twelve hundred a year. In the last two, or clinical, years the student was expected to be on the wards and to have seen the patients assigned to him, as well as to have performed the necessary laboratory work, before rounds at eight or nine o'clock. From then on he was busy throughout the day and into the evening. While this system had the advantage of providing maximal exposure to patients and clinical situations, it left little time for study.

Such a schedule was maintained despite the lack of availability of scholarship aid. Although by 1970 standards, tuition fees were exceedingly low—averaging $187 a year in 1922 [7]— the cost of a medical education was beyond the reach of students from low-income families unless they were both healthy and extremely dedicated. Very few schools had dormitories, but, as the schools were usually located in the poorer sections of large cities, cheap and often dingy accommodations were available nearby, and a student could earn his meals by waiting on table at a boarding house, and his room rent by stoking a furnace and sweeping stairs or by being in residence at an undertaker's establishment.

Most students at the time were from middle-class families of Western European ancestry: sons of physicians, clergymen, school teachers, small businessmen, and minor executives. Although racial or ethnic quotas were neither stated nor conceded, students with other backgrounds who made the grade had to possess unusual intellectual and personal qualities.[8]

Prior to the influx of older men in the postwar period, married students were almost unknown. The faculties considered wives to be unnecessary distractions, and married men, unless unusually well-qualified, were excluded from the better internships. This prejudice was not concealed—even graduates in the advanced stages of their residencies, at the age of twenty-eight to thirty, had to obtain their chiefs' permission to get married.

In the early years of the twentieth century, medical school student bodies included few women.[9] The Female Medical College of Pennsylvania, later known as the Woman's Medical College, and in 1970 as the Medical College of Pennsylvania, had been established in 1850 and for several decades was the major source of women physicians. Toward the end of the nineteenth century, western state universities were admitting women to the study of medicine, but it was not until 1893 that an eastern school, Johns Hopkins, accepted them on the same terms as men. The barriers were lowered at the University of Pennsylvania in 1914; at Yale and Columbia in 1917; and at most other schools over the next few years; Harvard held out until 1945.

Although theoretically eligible for admission, few women applied; in 1920 they constituted only 5.8 percent of the entering classes. College advisors discouraged all but the most determined, and at medical schools they were confronted in the deans' offices with such questions as: "Are you prepared to forego marriage and devote your entire life to medicine?" This situation was in sharp contrast to that in Europe where large numbers of women had for many years been admitted to the study of medicine.*

Medical school faculties were on many occasions criticized for the disproportion in the ratios of male and female students, but it seems fair to say that where prejudice existed it was expressed by failure to make positive efforts to recruit women rather than by lack of consideration for those who were strongly motivated enough to overcome the discouragement of their college advisors, families, and society in general. Year after year the percentage of female applicants accepted for admission was at least as high as that of male applicants.[10] The proportion of women admitted over the fifty-year period, 1920–70, increased gradually, reaching 9.6 percent in the entering classes in 1970. It was to increase further during the

---

* After World War II the percentage of women entering medicine in Western European countries ranged from 20 to 30; in Eastern Europe it was as high as 85.

following few years as the women's liberation movement gained momentum.

The attrition rate among women medical students was consistently higher than that for men. One study, covering the decade 1949–58, revealed a 15.51 percent dropout rate for women students and an 8.28 percent rate for men.[11] The difference was attributed primarily to nonacademic reasons.

The story of admission of black and other minority group students to medical schools was similar to that of women.[12,13] Following the Civil War several attempts were made to establish medical schools for blacks, but the weaker ones were forced to close and by 1920 only the two strongest, Meharry Medical College in Nashville, and the College of Medicine of Howard University in Washington, D.C., had survived.

Black students were admitted to medical schools in the North in limited numbers—actually the few who did apply and were qualified were given more than usual consideration. For economic and social reasons, and because many of those who attended college were enrolled at southern black colleges where educational standards were low, particularly in the sciences, few applicants could meet the minimal requirements. In 1938–39 only 1.64 percent of medical students were blacks, 87.1 percent of whom were enrolled in the two predominantly black schools. Little improvement in terms of percentage enrollment was to be observed over the next thirty years. In terms of numbers, however, enrollment increased by a multiple of three—from 350 to 1,042—and half of these students were in predominantly white schools. During this period there was a massive migration of rural black people to northern cities, where educational opportunities were more readily available and the civil rights movement was gaining strength.

The turning point for opportunities for members of minority groups, particularly blacks, to enter the medical profession occurred in about 1968. Stimulated by foundation support for advisory and recruitment programs, the predominantly white schools across the country opened their doors to minority students who could meet minimal academic requirements. The Josiah Macy, Jr. Foundation was to support such programs at thirty-six medical schools over the next few years. Other foundations, particularly the Commonwealth Fund and the Alfred Sloan Foundation, contributed large sums for distribution by National Medical Fellowships, Inc., thereby removing the financial barrier for hundreds of black students. Thus between 1968 and 1970 the number of blacks in entering classes increased sharply—from 266 to 697—and the percentage rose from 2.9 to 5.3. There was every indication that within the next few years the proportion of black medical students would approach that of the black population in the United States—then 11 percent.

FINANCIAL AID

During the period 1942–45, medical schools were in operation throughout the year on what was known as the "accelerated program." One nine-month academic year followed immediately after the other so that the four-year course could be completed in three years. Medical students and interns were deferred from active military service, but if physically qualified they were enrolled in the Army Specialized Training Corps or the Navy V-12 Program. They were relieved of payment of tuition fees, donned a uniform, drilled a few hours each week, and were subject to loose military discipline.

The G.I. Bill of Rights, enacted at the close of the war when the nation was exultant in victory and grateful to the returning veterans, opened up educational opportunities at all levels to hundreds of thousands of young men. Applications for admission to medical schools rose sharply, and their student bodies were soon composed of mature men who had experienced, or at least observed, suffering, homesickness, and danger, and had rubbed elbows with members of all social classes. They knew where they were going and what they wanted to do. Older faculty members agreed that they were, across the board, the best students they had ever known.

As eligibility for financial aid under the G.I. Bill was exhausted, scholarships became available from other sources.

Tuition fees rose sharply, and in the privately endowed universities reached a level of $2,500 to $3,000 by 1970. Medical education had become available to veterans of limited means, and some solution had to be found if it was not again to be confined largely to the offspring of the more affluent. The report, *Physicians for a Growing America,*[14] cited in Chapter XII as having had a major impact on other phases of medical education, revealed that 40 percent of the medical students enrolled in 1959 came from families with incomes of more than $10,000, although they constituted only 8 percent of families in the nation. Universities allocated more of their incomes to scholarships and made loans available; foundations and individuals contributed scholarship funds. Even so, medical students fared poorly compared to graduate students in other fields. In 1962–63, for example, 68 percent of students in graduate schools received nonrefundable grants averaging $2,450, while only 17 percent of medical students were so aided, and when they were their grants averaged only $585.[15] More assistance became available on passage of the Health Professions Educational Assistance Act of 1963, which provided grants to medical schools for both loans and scholarships to be distributed by the deans. By 1970, 44 percent of medical students were receiving some form of financial aid.

Examinations and Grades

In the 1920s and 1930s grades and class standings played important roles, with the result that the competitive attitude that prevailed among premedical students was carried over into the medical schools. In the preclinical years, particularly, there were frequent examinations during, and difficult examinations at the end of, each course. Class standings were determined by averaging course grades and, as they were of major importance in determining internship appointments at the better hospitals, even the best students were affected.

Students who failed one course were usually allowed to repeat the final examination at the end of the summer and, if successful, to advance with their classes. A summer course in gross anatomy offered at the University of Michigan saved the careers of many who later became successful physicians. Those who failed more than one course were required to repeat the year or withdraw. The attrition rate for all schools in the 1920s was approximately 25 percent over the four years, and highest in the first year. It was common practice for a dean to say to the entering class: "Look at the man on either side of you. A year from now one of them will be missing." As the selection process was improved, and examinations given less emphasis, the attrition rate decreased. In the 1960s dropouts over the four years of the course for all reasons amounted to less than 10 percent of the entering classes.

In retrospect it seems that the rigid examination system was undesirable and unnecessary for the large majority of intelligent and highly motivated students. While it may have forced some of the lazier students to study enough to get by, it encouraged the memorizing of details that were promptly forgotten after each examination. If the examinations of the National Board of Medical Examiners set at least minimal standards, as most medical educators believed they did, there were wide differences in the abilities of average students in the best and poorest schools, despite the pressure of local examinations. Without much doubt, many of those who flunked out of the schools with highest standards would have sailed through some of the poorer schools with flying colors.

The choice of an internship, and the competition for the limited number of positions in the popular hospitals, placed a severe strain on medical students during their senior years. They solicited letters of recommendation, filled out application forms, and travelled far and wide for interviews. Some hospitals even held written examinations. High-ranking students were offered places in hospitals of their second choice and were required to accept or reject such offers immediately, before knowing where they stood with their first choice. By 1950 approximately eight hundred hospitals were offering ten thousand approved internships to six thousand graduates.

In an effort to bring some order out of this chaos the

National Intern Matching Plan was established in 1951–52 as a joint program of the AAMC, AMA, and the hospital associations.[16,17] Under this plan the student listed the hospitals to which he had applied in his order of preference, and the hospitals listed the applicants in the order of their choice. The lists were then matched, and students and hospitals across the country were notified of the results simultaneously. After the bugs were worked out of the plan, and a few hospitals that resisted by offering places directly were brought into line, it was highly successful and was still in operation twenty years later.

Methods of Study

Over the years the average student's study methods changed less than most faculty members would have liked. As lectures decreased, so did the storage of copious notes to be regurgitated at the next examination. Group conferences and, in the clinical years, ward rounds replaced lectures. Students became better acquainted with medical journals, and when conscientious instructors provided specific references they often superseded textbooks. The latter, however, remained the standard fare because the volume of medical literature increased constantly and, except when involved in research or a special project, the search through the literature for relevant papers was too timeconsuming.

Audiovisual materials for individual study were introduced gradually in the postwar period, and the extent to which they were used depended largely on the quality of the slides, films, and film strips produced and the availability of equipment. Self-instructional and self-assessment material involving computer technology and the problem-oriented approach to patient evaluation and medical records were being used experimentally but had not come into common use in 1970.[18]

In spite of all these changes it cannot be said that medical students or their way of life were very different at the end of this half century than they were at the beginning. The students continued, by and large, to be serious, dedicated, hard-working, and, although sometimes beneath a tough exterior, compassionate. Physicians are accused of having lost interest in "the patient as a whole," an inevitable result of specialization, but that did not seem to me to be true of most medical students. As medical faculties became more research-oriented, many students followed the same pattern—but scientific interest and compassion are not incompatible. If any contrast is to be drawn, it seems fair to say that the average research-minded student in 1970 was more socially conscious than his clinically oriented counterpart in 1920.

NOTES

1. R. C. Lewis, "Methods of Admitting Medical Students," *Journal of Association of American Medical Colleges* 6 (1931): 17.

2. F. A. Moss, "Scholastic Aptitude Tests for Medical Students," *Journal of Association of American Medical Colleges* 6 (1931): 1.

3. W. Hale, "The Measurement of Medical Aptitude," *Journal of Association of American Medical Colleges* 21 (1946): 147.

4. J. M. Stalnaker, "Medical College Admissions Test," *Journal of Medical Education* 25 (1950): 428.

5. The problem of admissions practices is analyzed in detail in: *The Appraisal of Applicants to Medical Schools, Report of the Fourth Teaching Institute of the Association of American Medical Colleges* (Evanston, Illinois: Association of American Medical Colleges, 1957).

6. A. E. Severinghaus, H. J. Carman, and W. E. Cadbury, *Preparation for Medical Education in a Liberal Arts College* (New York: McGraw-Hill, 1953); and idem, *Preparation for Medical Education: A Restudy* (New York: McGraw-Hill, 1961).

7. D. F. Smiley, "History of the Association of American Medical Colleges, 1876–1956," *Journal of Medical Education* 32 (1957): 512.

8. For an extensive discussion of alleged discrimination in admissions, see: S. Jarcho, "Medical Education in the United States—1910–1956," *Journal of the Mount Sinai Hospital* 24 (July 1959): 339.

9. For a detailed account of women in medicine, and a bibliography on the subject, see: C. Lopate, *Women in Medicine* (Balti-

more: Johns Hopkins Press for the Josiah Macy, Jr. Foundation, 1968).

10. D. G. Johnson, "The Study of Applicants, 1964–65," *Journal of Medical Education* 40 (1965): 1026.

11. ——— "Doctor or Dropout? A Study of Medical Student Attrition," *Journal of Medical Education* 41 (1966): 1116.

12. D. C. Reitzes, *Negroes and Medicine* (Cambridge: Harvard University Press, 1958).

13. J. L. Curtis, *Blacks, Medical Schools, and Society* (Ann Arbor: University of Michigan Press, 1971).

14. The Surgeon General's Consultant Group on Medical Education, *Physicians for a Growing America* (Washington, D.C.: U.S. Government Printing Office, Public Health Services Publication No. 709, 1959).

15. "Datagrams: Medical School Application Trends for Classes Entering 1954–1965," *Journal of Medical Education* 40 (June 1965).

16. F. J. Mullin and J. M. Stalnaker, "The Matching Plan for Internship Appointment," *Journal of Medical Education* 26 (1951): 341.

17. J. M. Stalnaker, "The Matching Program for Intern Placement," *Journal of Medical Education* 28 (November 1953): 13.

18. L. L. Weed, *Medical Records, Medical Education and Patient Care* (Cleveland: Western Reserve University Press, 1969).

IV. From Graduation
to Professorship

I N the early years of the twentieth century the recent graduate who looked forward to becoming a professor in a clinical department started off as a rotating intern in a teaching hospital. Toward the end of a two-year rotation, he became house physician or surgeon and assumed many of the responsibilities later delegated to the chief resident. If he was fortunate, at the end of his internship he hung his shingle outside the office of an established practitioner.

While he had the privilege of caring for and collecting fees from his own patients, the demand for his services was seldom overwhelming and he assisted his mentor by making home visits, taking night calls, and doing simple laboratory work in the office, usually in lieu of paying office rent. It was to his advantage to spend as much time as possible in a teaching hospital as a junior attending physician or surgeon, working in the outpatient clinic several half-days a week, attending departmental meetings, and sometimes being privileged to make rounds or assist in the operating room.

As his practice grew and he became more competent, he opened his own office and became a full-fledged attending in the hospital. Those who were diligent in carrying out their clinical and teaching responsibilities would, after a few years, be appointed instructors in the medical school, and the most able moved up the academic ladder and eventually became clinical professors.

One can observe in this program the perpetuation of the apprenticeship system that prevailed a few decades earlier. The leaders in medical education who were responsible for introducing the full-time faculty and residency training systems were trained in this way. Many of them engaged in research and made important contributions without salaries, or the aid of grants, technical assistance, or even space beyond the corner of a bench in a pathology laboratory.

ACADEMIC PROGRESS PRIOR TO WORLD WAR II

Although the residency training and full-time faculty systems had been introduced late in the nineteenth century, they were adopted slowly. The Presbyterian Hospital in New York did not introduce residency training programs or appoint full-time faculty members as chiefs of services until 1928; the New York Hospital not until 1932.

Adoption of the full-time and residency systems resulted in a new kind of apprenticeship. The academically inclined graduate sought an internship appointment in a teaching hospital on a straight service, that is, he remained in one department throughout the year. He was given most of the routine responsibilities—admission histories, physical examinations, diagnostic procedures, parenteral treatments, and laboratory studies—that could not be delegated to the student clinical clerk. Then as now it was an exciting and satisfying experience. For the first time, the graduate had an opportunity to put into practice what he had learned, and he felt like a real doctor.

Interns and residents worked long hours, and the experience of remaining on duty over thirty-six hour periods with little or no sleep was generally accepted as one of the initiation rites associated with becoming a physician. Prior to World War II, when house officers were seldom married, they had to live in the hospital because room and board represented the major part of their compensation. They were theoretically off duty every other night and alternate weekends, but those who took full advantage of this privilege were considered loafers. In time, as more house officers married and as salaries increased, most of them lived outside and checked out during off-duty hours. Although older physicians looked on this custom as somewhat immoral, those in training continued to work a seventy- to one-hundred-hour week, while the average industrial worker was demanding a reduction of his thirty-six-hour-week schedule.

The pyramidal organization of the resident staff was well defined. Most services had two or three times as many interns as first-year residents, twice as many first- as second-year residents, and so on up the line until, after three to five years, the one survivor emerged as the chief resident. As such, he was a marked man: he had prestige, authority, and ready access to the professor. As the number of chief residents was limited by the small number of residency programs, a great many opportunities existed for these bright young men who had made the grade, and they stepped into instructorships without difficulty.

At this point they entered into another competition. As instructors they became assistant attendings on the services of teaching hospitals; took their turns on ward rounds and in operating rooms; worked in the outpatient clinics; taught medical students and nurses; and started to do independent research. Technical assistance was limited to the departmental *diener* who did everything from sweeping floors to repairing apparatus and caring for animals, usually assisted by an elderly woman who washed and sterilized the glassware. Research grants from outside sources were almost unknown and never available to the beginner; departmental research funds were distributed parsimoniously by the professor.

Advancement was slow in the 1920s, and perhaps even slower in the 1930s when the depression imposed reductions in staffs and a moratorium on promotions. Furthermore, promotions were dependent to a much greater extent than they were later on a balance of skills: one's ability as a clinician, teacher, and investigator. The customary period as an instructor was three to five years, as an assistant professor six years, and as an associate professor without tenure another five years. Real security was seldom reached before the age of forty. Most departments had only one professor who remained chairman of the department until he retired or died.

Certainly no one remained in academic medicine in those days for the financial rewards. Interns were provided with board, room, and laundry services, but no stipend. Assistant residents were paid from $400 to $800 per year, and chief residents up to $1,000. Instructors' and assistant professors' salaries were in the range of $2,400 to $4,000, and as late as 1940 distinguished professors received only $10,000 to $15,000. By 1970, interns were being paid almost as much as that.

In the pre–World War II era, full-time faculties, although few in number, gradually took over from the part-time faculty members the lectures, ward rounds, and conferences. The typical teacher remained a generalist within his specialty; the senior surgeon operated for every condition from brain tumors to intestinal perforations; and the internist in charge of a ward service supervised the treatment of all patients admitted, and only occasionally consulted another member of his department who had similar responsibility for a ward service but a special interest in a particular facet of internal medicine, such as cardiology or metabolism.

Post–World War II

After World War II, the forces that were influential in fragmenting the basic science disciplines acted on the clinical disciplines in a similar manner. Full-time faculties expanded rapidly, and faculty members became more specialized in their clinical and research interests, and consequently in their teaching activities. By 1970 a respectable department of surgery or medicine had to include ten or a dozen subspecialty sections, each with its chief, junior faculty members, residents, and fellows.

The system of residency training also changed. Rotating internships became less popular and were gradually abandoned by the teaching hospitals. The senior student made a crucial career decision when he applied for a straight internship that confined his activity to a single discipline. Medical interns were assigned to various inpatient and outpatient services for periods of a few months, and they participated in the care of patients with a cross-section of nonsurgical illnesses. In the same manner, surgical interns were assigned to the several surgical subspecialties or general surgical wards where they took part in pre- and postoperative care and assisted at operations for a variety of conditions.

The surgeon who did every type of operation was gradually replaced by the subspecialist, and the residents followed the same course, so that after his internship the young surgeon became an assistant resident in what was called "general surgery" (largely abdominal surgery), urology, orthopedics, otolaryngology, or one of the other surgical specialties. Similarly, the assistant medical resident had the opportunity to elect a special field of interest, although the medical service was less fragmented than the surgical field. A by-product of this change was a breakdown in the highly competitive pyramidal system that had prevailed previously, as a larger number of residents rose to senior posts in one or another subspecialty.

In the medical field, particularly, the tendency to subspecialization was reinforced by the availability of postdoctoral fellowships financed by grants from the federal government, notably the National Institutes of Health. These training grants, awarded to the medical schools by the NIH in the form of fellowship stipends and some faculty salaries, were intended originally to prepare young physicians for careers in clinical investigation. In time the awards became so numerous and so readily available that they also fostered the development of a corps of subspecialists in private practice.

In some university hospitals, fellows outnumbered residents—with resulting conflicts. Although theoretically the resident staff was responsible for patient care, the resident often found a fellow in cardiology or gastroenterology interposed between him and the patient. As the staffs of residents and fellows increased, educational programs for trainees became more formal, and grand rounds, clinical-pathological and radiological conferences, research seminars, and similar activities occupied a considerable amount of the fellows' time and as many hours as the residents could spare from clinical work.

In terms of education, the fellowship programs had many virtues. For the young physician, whose every minute had been occupied throughout four years in medical school, a year of internship, and two or three years of residency, a year or two under less pressure with time for study and research was a refreshing experience. These fellowship programs produced many of the most competent teachers, investigators, and practitioners in the subspecialties.

The impact of federal subsidies for residency training was especially apparent in the field of psychiatry. Perhaps there would have been public concern for mental health even if there had been no war, but World War II did emphasize the need for physicians trained to care for psychoneuroses. A crash program to increase the production of psychiatrists was stimulated by the award by the NIH of large numbers of fellowships that provided salaries for psychiatric residents well above the level of those paid to residents in other disciplines. This program was in operation for approximately twenty years, and it was not until the late 1960s, when the salary scale for all residents was improved, that residents in psychiatry ceased to be a privileged group.

THE BASIC MEDICAL SCIENCES

There were fewer changes in the preclinical departments during the 1920s and 1930s. The impact of the Flexner Report had resulted in the establishment of full-time basic science faculties who had heavy teaching responsibilities in the medical curriculum, few graduate students, and limited technical assistance and research facilities. It was possible to be promoted and to live a satisfying life as a teacher, with little pretense of being an investigator.

Many preclinical departments had extensive clinical responsibilities: departments of biochemistry and bacteriology performed routine diagnostic examinations for teaching hospitals; the performance and interpretation of electrocardiograms and basal metabolism tests were often the responsibilities of departments of physiology; departments of pathology, then as later, did autopsies and surgical pathology. As full-time physicians were appointed in clinical departments, one after another of the laboratory diagnostic procedures were taken over by the clinicians. Hematologists in departments of medicine and pediatrics became the experts on examination of the cellular elements in blood; metabolists relieved the biochemists of responsibility for chemical examinations; specialists in infectious diseases set up their own bacteriology laboratories; and so on, until the basic scientists were relieved entirely of duties related to patient care. The third stage was the consolidation of all laboratory diagnostic procedures, with the usual exception of surgical pathology, in a central department of laboratory medicine or clinical pathology under the management of the teaching hospital.

It is difficult to assign dates to the steps in this evolution because the changes took place almost imperceptibly and at different times in various institutions. It can only be said that in 1920 the basic scientists often had a close relationship on a service basis with their nearby teaching hospitals, and that by 1960 that relationship no longer existed. Two exceptions to this generalization must be mentioned: the departments of pathology and pharmacology, which are usually considered bridge departments rather than preclinical or clinical, continued to have a dual role; in fact the emergence of clinical pharmacology as a subspecialty strengthened the clinical relationship.

The impact of these changes on the teaching programs of medical schools and the attitudes of basic science faculties was greater than is generally recognized. In the 1920s the basic sciences were taught by individuals who, although often not physicians, had an interest in clinical medicine and made an effort to relate their instruction to clinical problems. As they were relieved of clinically related responsibilities they turned their attention to more fundamental issues. The anatomists lost interest in gross anatomy as it related to surgery and became electron microscopists and cellular biologists; the biochemists turned from nutrition and intermediary metabolism to molecular structure and enzymology, and the physiologists from the function of mammalian organ systems to cells; the bacteriologists became microbiologists concerned with microbial physiology and genetics; and the pharmacologists turned from studying the effect of drugs on intact animals to chemistry and the effect of chemical agents at the cellular level.

From the standpoint of the advancement of medical science these were logical developments, and the results were impressive. The infusion of federal subsidies in the form of research and training grants led to the rapid expansion of basic science faculties and a diminished teaching load for individual faculty members. Furthermore, as they became more specialized, instruction became more fragmented. Student reaction to these developments was generally unfavorable. Although the material presented was of great scientific interest, too little effort was made to emphasize its relevance to clinical problems.

Social and Economic Consequences

For both basic science and clinical faculties these changes in the training programs and the increased emphasis on research had social and economic consequences. As faculties expanded, as new schools opened, and as federal grants for support of research became more available, competition for the services of the more talented investigators intensified and faculty members became more mobile—the average faculty member moved from one institution to another two or three times during his career. Furthermore, there were subtle and not altogether desirable changes in the qualifications for promotion. Although the regulations continued to state that competence in teaching and research should be weighed equally, the volume of research publications all too frequently became the dominating factor in determining advancement.

There were also subtle changes in the value system. With the influx of federal funds in the 1950s and 1960s, salary scales improved and the differential between the incomes, after taxes, of full-time faculty members and practitioners became less pronounced. In general, those in the surgical specialties had higher incomes than internists and pediatricians, and clinicians were paid a quarter to a third more than basic scientists. Even so, basic medical scientists were usually on a higher salary scale than the faculties of arts and sciences, and when the medical school was on the university campus this discrepancy became the source of a controversy that was seldom resolved. In many institutions a solution was found by having the medical faculty employed on an eleven-months-a-year basis, with a one-month vacation, while other faculties had the privilege of longer vacations.

Money became a less important factor in attracting faculty members from one institution to another, and the provision of facilities became a more decisive consideration. Bargaining was often on the basis of square feet of laboratory space rather than dollars, and the preservation or expansion of space assigned to a department or one of its subdivisions was often the determining factor in the retention or loss of a valuable faculty member.

In the days of part-time faculties, recruitment was almost entirely local, and the large urban medical schools had the great advantage of substantial reservoirs of talent. In the 1920s the two principal sources of full-time faculties were Johns Hopkins and the Rockefeller Institute for Medical Research. Older schools such as Yale and the University of Virginia, which were reorganized, and new schools such as Vanderbilt, Rochester, and Duke, which were founded at that time in smaller cities, were consequently influenced extensively by the Hopkins customs and attitudes. Schools in the larger cities were more self-sufficient and, except where there was extensive reorganization and the construction of new medical centers, faculty positions were more often filled locally.

As full-time faculties expanded, new schools opened, and research activity increased, there were more sources of well-qualified faculty members, and finding just the right person to fill a vacancy became more difficult. When a tenured position, particularly a departmental chairmanship, was to be filled, although extensive inquiries were made at other schools, the ideal candidate could easily be overlooked. In the late 1950s an effort was made to have vacancies announced in the *Journal of Medical Education,* but the plan was not accepted generally and was abandoned after a few years. This unorganized system of recruitment, although outmoded, still existed in 1970. In the opinion of many it should have been replaced by the European system of public announcement under which anyone who considers himself eligible may indicate his availability in a dignified and acceptable manner by submitting his curriculum vitae and bibliography.

In summary, over these fifty years there was a remarkable change in the career development of a faculty member. Instead of starting out as a generalist in a broad field of medicine he became committed to a narrow field of specialization early in his career. Research became an increasingly important factor in determining his progress. Although the period of training for clinicians was lengthened, economic security was attained earlier. Movement in and out of the academic circle became more difficult.

V. Faculty Organization and Governance[1]

E ARLY in the twentieth century, medical faculties were loosely organized bodies not requiring, or at least surviving without, much administration. Most of the schools had developed independently or with a loose affiliation with their parent universities. Faculties were composed largely of practicing physicians who carried out their academic responsibilities voluntarily or with minimal compensation.

THE DEANSHIP

The deans were of two types: most were senior practitioners chosen because they occupied positions of prestige in the community; others were chosen from among the few basic scientists. They could occupy this position without serious interference with other activities, as their duties consisted largely of presiding over occasional faculty meetings and graduation exercises. A sign that hung outside the dean's office at Yale School of Medicine in 1910 read: "Office Hours. 8:30-9:30 a.m. Wednesdays."

As more full-time faculty members were hired, the dean was usually chosen from among that group, but the center of his activities remained in his department and he dropped into the dean's office only occasionally. The day-to-day business was conducted by a faithful secretary who served as registrar, bookkeeper, and custodian, as well as counselor to and disciplinarian of the students.

Even the largest medical schools were administered under this arrangement, although with diminishing success as their problems became more complicated. During his first five years as dean of the Harvard Medical School, David Edsell was also chief of the medical service at the Massachusetts General Hospital. It was not until 1923 that he moved the base of his operations to the medical school and became one of the first full-time medical deans in the United States.[2]

Throughout the half-century considered in this report the role of the dean continued to be controversial and often ill-defined, differing of course with the local situation and the personality of the incumbent.

Until the end of World War II the deanship was a comparatively comfortable position to which many faculty members aspired. The problems encountered were relatively uncomplicated and external pressures were minimal. Funds, although limited, were derived from internal sources, and it was the dean's responsibility to see that they were distributed in such a manner as to encourage high standards and a balanced operation. His concerns were academic and related largely to the faculty, students, and curriculum. Although most deanships had become full-time obligations, to the extent that the incumbents withdrew from practice and departmental chairmanships, they still found time for some teaching, clinical activities, or research, and most of them had few responsibilities at the national level. With the aid of a part-time assistant dean, who usually dealt with admissions and student affairs, a dean could handle the job without being overwhelmed.

In the postwar period this situation changed dramatically. A major force was the expansion of research activities resulting from the growing availability of funds for that purpose, unaccompanied by a corresponding rise in general institutional support. Grants for research projects and programs led to an unbalanced expansion of departments and activities within them, without regard to the requirements of teaching programs or the general welfare of the institution. In an effort to keep pace with the demand for research facilities and a rapidly rising salary scale, the dean's attention was diverted to fund-raising and justification of expanding capital and operating budgets.

For those medical schools affiliated with universities, relationships with the central administration and other university divisions continued to be complicated, and communication between the dean, as the spokesman for the school, and the president's office was difficult. This was particularly true in the latter half of the period under review, when the budget of the medical center was often half as large as that for the remainder of the university. If the dean did not have the authority to manage the institution for which he was responsible his administration was doomed to failure, and yet he was obliged to operate within the policies of the university.

An unfortunate result of these social, economic, and financial strains was that the medical school administration lost its stability. While the deanship was seldom, and should not be, a lifetime job, the rapid turnover in the dean's office experienced by many schools led to inefficiency and a deterioration of morale. The kinds of people who had been the best deans were those who gained considerable satisfaction from the achievements of those they supported, directly or indirectly. But as the degree of frustration exceeded the yield of satisfaction the deans became discouraged. While during the decade 1949–59 there were eleven new deans in eighty-two medical schools, there were sixty-seven new deans in the same schools during the decade 1959–69. The average tenure decreased from seven to four years.

The complexity of financial management was magnified during the 1960s as total expenditures for medical schools increased from $400 million to $1.5 billion. In the well-organized dean's office the accountant became the most essential staff member. Other functions such as admissions and student affairs, community relations, continuing education, and hospital relationships were delegated to associate deans.

During the postwar period, as the academic medical center emerged, many of the housekeeping and extramural activities were taken over by the medical center administration.

Departmental Organization

The administrative structure within the schools also underwent a substantial change during this period. In 1920 the basic science departments consisted of anatomy, biochemistry (or physiological chemistry), physiology, pathology, bacteriology, and pharmacology. (Physiology and pharmacology were sometimes combined.) A department seldom had more than a half-dozen full-time members. The most common clinical departments were medicine, surgery, pediatrics, and obstetrics and gynecology. In some schools other specialties such as urology and orthopedics had departmental status; departments of psychiatry and radiology usually appeared later.

Clinical departments were staffed largely by practicing physicians, and were located in one or more hospitals operated quite independently of the medical school. In some instances the association hinged on a faculty member's personal control of a hospital service, and its availability for teaching on his goodwill. Although individual faculty members could be as recalcitrant as they are today, departments lacked the size and cohesion that made them as powerful, and at times as seriously disturbing to the equanimity and productivity of the schools, as they became later.

The problems of management caused by the rapid growth in size and complexity of the operation were not confined to the dean's office. As departments expanded they tended to become fragmented, and direct communication between the department head and individual faculty members was diminished. In the early part of this period, members of a department had common interests; their offices and laboratories were located off a single corridor and they talked with each other daily. As each of the senior members, aided by teaching and research grants, gathered around him a corps of junior faculty members, fellows, and technicians, departmental cohesion was reduced.

In the basic sciences the formal administrative structure usually remained unchanged, although the groups functioned more or less independently. In the clinical departments, however, there was constant pressure to establish new and independent units, fostered by the clinical specialty societies and encouraged by the subdivision of the specialty boards. The administrations of some universities succumbed to this pressure, and schools that had operated with a dozen departments found themselves with twice that number. Others compromised by establishing semiautonomous sections such as urology, otolaryngology, and orthopedics within the department of surgery, and neurology, dermatology, hematology, and metabolism within the department of medicine.

The cohesion of the departments was further disturbed by the disappearance of clearly defined borders between the disciplines. Cardiac physiologists found that they had more in common with clinical cardiologists and cardiac surgeons than with neurophysiologists in their own departments.

Departmental chairmen, like the deans, became overwhelmed with administrative duties and less able to maintain their competence as clinicians and scientists. Those who were well adjusted and realistic delegated some administrative functions to other faculty members, and in a few schools the pressure was relieved by appointment of capable administrative assistants. For many, however, the prestige and authority vested in these positions was not sufficiently attractive to compensate for the loss of their opportunity to function professionally. From the standpoints of both the chairman and the institution, it became apparent that the appointment of chairmen with indefinite administrative tenure was no longer a satisfactory arrangement. In some universities the appointments of all administrative officers, including deans and chairmen, were for a defined period, subject to review and to renewal if mutually satisfactory at the end of that time.

Faculty Organization

Without doubt, medical faculties met periodically from the time the schools were founded, and the records of their deliberations are available in many schools. These meetings had more to do with awarding degrees and with student affairs than with governance, however. By 1920 the faculties had grown in size and were departmentalized enough to require some kind of coordinating body, which usually took the form of a committee of department heads, sometimes supplemented by elected members, known as an executive committee. In addition to routine functions such as recommendations for the award of degrees and faculty promotions and appointments, these committees soon became the policy-making bodies for the schools. This concentration of power in an oligarchy of departmental chairmen had its good and bad features: on the one hand, it encouraged cooperation, concern for the school as a whole, and balanced development; on the other, it deprived the majority of faculty members of any voice, and had the potential to overpower a less-than-forceful dean.

By the 1960s the demand of junior faculty and students for more influence, or at least representation, had become more vociferous—and many schools responded either by changing the composition of the executive committees to include more elected members, or by establishing parallel committees known as senates or councils. In both instances, while the result was a more cumbersome system of governance, there were certain advantages.

Although disturbing to the older and more conservative faculty members, the introduction of young blood had its good effects. The research programs fueled by federal funds often dominated the attention of the faculty, who seemed to forget that the medical school's fundamental mission was to teach medical students. The presence of students on curriculum committees, and their overt criticism of teaching methods and the performance of some of their instructors, helped to bring about a better distribution of faculty energy.

Faculty Practice and Compensation

As long as the clinical departments were staffed by practicing physicians, their compensation, if any, and their institutional competition with the independent practitioners presented no serious problems. By 1920, however, the trend to appoint full-time clinical faculties was gaining momentum and universities were assuming greater responsibility for operating university-owned or closely affiliated hospitals.

If they were to remain competent, full-time teachers of clinical medicine had to take personal responsibility for the care of at least a few private patients, even though this activity did not supplement their incomes. These few patients did not affect the teaching program to any extent because the wards and outpatient clinics were well supplied with indigent patients who were cared for by the resident staffs under the guidance of attending physicians. As insurance plans were introduced and more people became eligible for treatment by private physicians, with their fees being paid by third parties, the ward populations began to shrink. Private patients became important from the standpoint of education, and the collection of fees for the services of full-time faculty members became a significant source of income.

These developments introduced new administrative problems. To what extent should the medical school control the private practice of its full-time clinical faculty, and what should be the disposition of the income generated? These questions were approached by the schools in a variety of ways, ranging from total institutional control of private practice, and the income derived therefrom, to complete freedom. At one end of the spectrum were the strict full-time faculty members whose salaries were paid by the university or affiliated hospital, and whose status and fringe benefits were the same as those of faculty members elsewhere in the university. Fees from practice were turned over to the school, and any salary supplement paid as a reward for participation in practice was modest in amount and controlled by institutional policy. At the other end of the spectrum were the geographical full-time faculty members whose professional activities were based in the medical school or teaching hospital, and who were paid only partial salaries from basic university sources. They received additional income from private practice.

Where fees were paid directly to the faculty member, with no institutional control, the situation usually got completely out of hand and had to be corrected. On the other hand, in the absence of financial incentive, faculty members were less likely to be productive financially in caring for private patients, and the school lost seriously needed income. They were often careless about reporting clinical services rendered and indifferent to the necessity of making the appropriate charges.

Most schools eventually adopted some form of compromise between the strict full-time system and uncontrolled practice. A ceiling was placed on income derived from practice, and any excess reverted to the department or to the school or was divided between them.

Where the department was the primary beneficiary there were inevitable consequences. Surgeons had the opportunity to make large amounts, while pediatricians, at the other end of the scale, found it difficult to supplement their incomes or contribute to the departmental budget. Consequently there were rich and poor clinical departments and inadequately supported basic science departments. Another undesirable aspect of this arrangement was that departments became more independent of the dean's office, and the governing relationship between the departments and the dean was altered substantially.

By 1970 the whole problem of financing medical education remained unresolved, and the extent to which the schools would be dependent on income from the care of patients by their faculties was difficult to predict. With a decline in ward services, active participation in the care of patients capable of paying professional fees, either directly or through governmental or voluntary insurance plans, was essential to the maintenance of teaching programs. It seemed likely that no satisfactory solution would be found until a national program for the provision of health services was established.

Over the half century under consideration, many medical schools experienced a considerable disintegration in the sense of academic community. Student enrollment rose gradually, with periods of acceleration during 1942–45 and 1962–70. As research activity flourished in the postwar era, however, faculties increased disproportionately. Faculty members became more mobile and, with much of the support for salaries and facilities coming from outside sources, there was a decline in their sense of loyalty—if conditions were not to their liking, groups of investigators, supported by program grants amounting to hundreds of thousands of dollars, could pack up and move to another institution.

University–Hospital Relationships

The governance problems of medical schools were not entirely intramural. The maintenance of balanced relationships with both their universities and their communities, as well as their educational, research, and service roles, was not an easy task.[3]

From time to time the existence of strong basic medical science departments was threatened by the desire of biologists in faculties of arts and science to expand their spheres of influence. As molecular biology developed and the biologists became increasingly concerned with the study of fundamental life processes, some of them looked on medical scientists as contaminating "pure" biology by less than precise application of the science to such complicated and uncontrollable subjects as humans. They proposed to take over instruction and research in the basic medical sciences, except pathology and pharmacology, and leave to the medical faculties the mundane task of vocational training.

To those involved in medical education and research such proposals were ridiculous. They became even more impractical as preclinical and clinical teaching were integrated, and as efforts were made to base instruction in the diagnosis and treatment of disease on an understanding of underlying alterations in structure and function, rather than on memorization of signs and symptoms and standard therapies. Furthermore, the quality of medical research was dependent on easy communication and collaboration among basic and clinical scientists.

The medical scientists were well aware of the desirability of a close relationship among the medical and other divisions of the university, including the social and natural sciences. They also realized that the tools of medicine include urinals and emesis basins as well as computers and mass spectro-photometers. The capacity to straddle the line between theory and practicality placed medical schools among the most productive institutions in our society.

Relationships with affiliated hospitals continued to be sources of intermittent conflict. In some instances the hospital, as the wealthier of the partners, was in a position to dictate the educational policies and administration of the medical school. Conversely, when the hospital was owned and operated by the university or was financially dependent on it, the resources of the medical school were drained to support service programs. The petty details of allocation of space and expenses were often causes of friction. At many academic medical centers these conflicts were diminished by the establishment of joint administrative boards composed of officers and trustees of the two institutions.

In summary, the governance of medical schools changed over this period from a free-and-easy system based on the intimacy and devotion of small cohesive groups, meagerly supported by local funds, to a complex system requiring a variety of management skills and a highly organized administrative structure. In the face of an accelerating demand for universities to play more active public service roles, there was little evidence in 1970 that administrators of medical schools could look forward to a more comfortable future.

NOTES

1. In parts of this chapter I have drawn heavily on: *Report of the Commission for the Study of the Governance of the Academic Medical Center* (New York: Josiah Macy, Jr. Foundation, 1970).

2. J. C. Aub and R. K. Hapgood, *Pioneer in Modern Medicine: David Linn Edsall of Harvard* (Cambridge: Harvard Medical Alumni Association, 1970).

3. V. W. Lippard, "The Medical School—Janus of the University," *Journal of Medical Education* 30 (1955): 698.

VI. The Rise of Academic Medical Centers

THE program of medical education in the United States had its roots in the British system, which was dominated by the hospital schools of London, and the German system, in which medical studies were centered in the universities. The first American schools were founded by colleges that were later to become universities. Others were subsequently established by the staffs of hospitals,* or, in the case of proprietary schools, without any institutional base. Academic medical centers represent a fusion of the British and German systems in that they combine the resources of a hospital, or group of hospitals, and a university. Their organization during the fifty-year period under review is of great significance in the history of medical education.

It was customary for medical schools located in large cities to make arrangements for clinical instruction in municipal or voluntary hospitals, many of which were situated at some distance from the schools and were operated independently, that is, the schools assumed no direct responsibility for the hospitals' administration or finances.† As schools were established on university campuses, particularly at state institutions located in rural areas, the establishment of associated teaching hospitals became essential. They were owned and operated by the universities and financed with state funds.‡

---

* Hospital schools appeared in the 1860s with the founding of the Bellevue Medical College in New York City and the Long Island College of Medicine in Brooklyn.

† An example of such a relationship that still exists is that of the Harvard Medical School and several Boston hospitals.

‡ Examples of such arrangements are the medical schools and associated university hospitals at the universities of Virginia, Michigan, and Iowa.

The formation of academic medical centers by merging university medical schools and several urban hospitals represented a different approach. Under this arrangement the several institutions assumed joint responsibility for providing education, research, and service in one location. This pattern is illustrated by the organization of the Columbia–Presbyterian and New York Hospital–Cornell medical centers in New York City in the 1920s.

The Columbia–Presbyterian Medical Center

The College of Physicians and Surgeons of Columbia University had been one of the leading medical schools in the United States since it was founded in 1767.* During its first 161 years it depended for clinical instruction on various hospitals that permitted members of the faculty to teach in their wards and clinics. This arrangement was considered unsatisfactory in many ways, and the desirability of establishing a general hospital under university auspices was mentioned repeatedly in reports of the university's deans and presidents.

Influenced by the Flexner Report, in 1910 Edward S. Harkness, financier, philanthropist, and benefactor of the Commonwealth Fund, wrote letters to the governing boards of the Presbyterian Hospital and of Columbia University in which he outlined a plan for affiliation, backed up with an offer of substantial financial assistance. Among the conditions of this proposed gift was an understanding that the wards and clinics of the hospital would be available for teaching medical students, and that the staff would be nominated by the university. A formal agreement between the two institutions was signed a year later, and development of the complex that was to be known as the Columbia–Presbyterian Medical Center was initiated.

* It was founded as the Medical Faculty of King's College, which later became Columbia College, and subsequently Columbia University. The medical faculty was merged with the College of Physicians and Surgeons, organized independently by the Medical Society of the County of New York in 1807.

Memoranda and revisions of the agreement followed, one after another, over the following fifteen years.[1] In the meantime, the disadvantages of isolation and the value of a close association with a university and a general hospital with strong medical and surgical services became apparent to several specialty hospitals. The Sloane Hospital for Women and the Vanderbilt Clinic, formerly operated by Columbia, were incorporated in the center, as were Babies Hospital and the Neurological Institute. Negotiations with the state of New York led to construction of the New York State Psychiatric Institute and Hospital on land provided by the medical center, and it became an integral unit. Plans were completed, and ground was broken in 1925; the medical center was opened three years later.

The New York Hospital–Cornell Medical Center

The Cornell University Medical College was founded in 1898 in New York City, over two hundred miles from its parent university. The preclinical departments were located in Ithaca and also across the street from Bellevue Hospital, a municipal institution operated by the city of New York. The college was also affiliated with the New York Hospital, the Lying-in Hospital, the New York Nursery and Child's Hospital, the Memorial Hospital, and others. The students travelled by subway from one hospital to another, and the hospitals had little connection with each other or with the preclinical departments.

From the standpoint of the medical college there was an obvious need for consolidation of its physical plant in close association with a major teaching hospital where its activities could be centralized. The officers of the New York Hospital, founded in 1771—the oldest hospital in New York and second oldest in the colonies—looked favorably on an opportunity to play a larger role in teaching and research. After negotiations extending over several years a formal agreement was signed in 1927. The preamble of the agreement stated that:

. . . the Hospital is impressed with the importance of rendering a larger and more important service to the sick of the community and to medical science through a more intimate and organic association with the Medical College. . . . The University wishes to associate itself organically with the Hospital . . . for the purpose of developing the Medical School on advanced and steadily advancing university lines. In the teaching of students and in the development of medical research it is the common purpose of the two institutions to be in a position to offer opportunities which will attract to the staff and faculty the ablest teachers, investigators and physicians that are anywhere procurable.[2]

The agreement went on to stipulate that while the two institutions would maintain their corporate identities, their activities would be coordinated through a joint administrative board. The most important consideration was that they would not merely operate side by side, one concerned with service and the other with teaching and research, but would be mutually concerned with all three functions.

The Lying-in Hospital and the New York Nursery and Child's Hospital were merged with the hospital–medical school complex and their resources contributed to the construction and operation of the obstetric and pediatric clinics.

Three city blocks on the East River were acquired. A twenty-four-story building, incorporating the patient care units and outpatient clinics of the hospital and classrooms and laboratories of the college, was erected on one block, and the nurses' residence, power plant, and supporting services on the others. Forty years later this majestic structure was still one of the most beautiful buildings in New York City.[3]

A full-time faculty of eminent physicians and scientists was assembled. A resident training program was introduced under the leadership of a group of chief residents who had served in similar capacities at other teaching hospitals.

The medical center came to life as the first patient was admitted on September 5, 1932, by which time the economic depression that followed the collapse of the stock market in 1929 was well advanced. Most of the resources that had originally been considered adequate for both construction and operation of the complex had been expended for construction, and the center had a difficult time financially over the next decade. Salaries and departmental budgets were reduced, and the sense of insecurity that prevailed led to a decline in the morale of the faculty. The center weathered the depression, however, and became one of the country's leading centers of medical care, education, and research.

DEVELOPMENT OF OTHER CENTERS

The founding of these two great medical centers set a pattern that was followed, with many variations, throughout the country over the next several decades. It was recognized that the day of the isolated specialty hospital had passed, and that the highest quality of medical care could be provided, and teaching and research accomplished most efficiently, when the resources of medical schools and hospitals were combined. As new schools were founded, the classrooms, libraries, and research laboratories were integrated structurally and functionally with clinical facilities for patient care.* Older schools and their associated teaching hospitals reorganized their physical plants and administrative structures in a similar manner.† This trend was further advanced by plans for new health professional education centers developed in the 1960s in which teaching hospitals and schools of medicine, dentistry, nursing, allied health professions, pharmacy, and social services were located in one setting.

It is not surprising that it was to the academic medical centers that patients who required diagnostic and therapeutic facilities and specialized skills not available in community hospitals were referred. Consequently, the centers became the focal points of Regional Medical Programs. In a report published in 1970 the Carnegie Commission on Higher Education recommended that the centers assume a similar role in the initial and continuing education of all types of health

---

* Examples are Duke University (1930); the University of California, Los Angeles (1951); and the University of Florida (1956).
† Examples are Yale, Northwestern, and Stanford universities.

personnel.[4] Satellite units, to be known as "area health education centers," located in community hospitals would conduct educational programs with the guidance of the faculties of the university centers.

Academic medical centers made possible the geographic, functional, and administrative integration of several institutions for the purpose of providing the highest type of education, research, and patient care. They were dedicated to the concept that this goal is most likely to be attained by the center as a whole than by the constituent units acting separately. The wisdom of this concept has been demonstrated over the years when one compares the achievements and efficiency of operation of the well-integrated centers with those in which several hospitals and a medical school have been built on one plot of ground but have remained independent— structurally and administratively.

NOTES

1. The several agreements and revisions adopted from time to time are recorded, along with a history of the Columbia–Presbyterian Medical Center, in: W. C. Rappleye, *The Current Era of the Faculty of Medicine, Columbia University, 1910–1958* (New York: Columbia University Press, 1958).

2. A detailed account of this merger, and the early history of the New York Hospital–Cornell Medical College association, may be found in: G. C. Robinson, *Adventures in Medical Education* (Cambridge: Harvard University Press, 1957).

3. For a poetic tribute to this building, see: H. E. Sigerist, *American Medicine* (New York: Norton, 1934).

4. Carnegie Commission on Higher Education, *Higher Education and the Nation's Health* (New York: McGraw-Hill, 1970).

VII. The Veterans Hospitals[1]

IT has been said that the three influences that had the most telling effect on medical education in the twentieth century were the Flexner Report, the entry of the federal government into the support of medical research, and the establishment of a close relationship between veterans hospitals and their neighboring medical schools. Inclusion of the veterans hospital–medical school relationship in a category with the other two factors is only a slight exaggeration of its importance.

Participation of the federal government in the provision of medical care dates back to 1798, when the Congress passed "an act for the relief of sick and disabled seamen." Marine hospitals have continued to operate at various ports in the United States since that time, although they have never played an important role in medical education. Parallel to the organization of a federally supported service for seamen there was recognition of public responsibility for those disabled in the military services. The initial approach to provision of medical care was indirect and incidental to domiciliary care. A home for "disabled and decrepit naval officers, seamen and marines" was opened in Philadelphia in 1833, and two similar institutions for invalid and disabled soldiers were in operation before the Civil War. Legislation was enacted in 1865 to establish the National Asylum for Disabled Volunteer Soldiers, and the first of these homes was opened in Togus, Maine, in 1866.

With America's entry into World War I came the first legislative assignment to the federal government of responsibility for furnishing medical benefits to veterans, as distinguished from domiciliary care. This responsibility was at first met haphazardly by the admission of disabled veterans to marine hospitals, army and navy hospitals, and soldiers' homes.

The United States Veterans Bureau was established in 1921, and the administration of medical and hospital services for veterans was transferred from the Public Health Service to this new agency. Other functions pertaining to veterans, such as administration of pensions and some of the domiciliary facilities, remained under other federal departments until consolidated under the reorganized Veterans Administration (VA) in 1930.

The Veterans Bureau took over forty-seven institutions, few of which could legitimately be termed hospitals, in 1922. Over the following twenty years the number increased to ninety-one. Many of these institutions were located in isolated areas where they could maintain little communication with modern medical facilities. Furthermore, recruitment of physicians was inhibited by the rigidity of the civil service, low salaries, poor equipment, and little opportunity for research or for continuing education.

During the period between the two world wars the controversy over admission to veterans hospitals of patients with non-service-connected disabilities was gradually resolved. Bed capacity was increased beyond the demand for care of service-connected illnesses, and at first the vacant beds were filled by veterans with neuropsychiatric disorders and tuberculosis. Later, veterans were admitted with non-service-connected disabilities that would otherwise have been cared for in acute general hospitals. By 1941, 78 percent of the patients were being treated for illnesses not associated with military service.

The end of World War II found the VA hospitals poorly equipped or staffed to care for the 13 million members of the armed forces being returned to civilian life. Together with veterans of earlier wars, 17 million persons were at that time eligible for care.

A major incident leading to the change in character of VA medical programs was the meeting of the House of Delegates of the American Medical Association in December 1945. The man who spoke for the VA was its new chief medical director, Major General Paul R. Hawley, formerly chief surgeon of the European Theatre of Operations (ETO). A physician with almost three decades of regular military service, he was outspoken and emotional in his appeal to the medical profession and the medical schools to help him bring the system of veterans hospitals into the mainstream of American medicine. General Hawley contended that the uninspired corps of civil service physicians previously employed should be replaced by specialty-board-certified physicians returning from military service. Backing him were such prominent figures as Fred W. Rankin, professor of surgery at the University of Minnesota, and Elliot C. Cutler, professor of surgery at Harvard, who had served with him in the ETO.

The man credited with having drafted the concrete plan for reorganizing the staffs of the VA hospitals is Paul B. Magnuson, professor of orthopedic surgery at Northwestern University. For civilian medical officers, whose training had been interrupted by the war, residencies would be established in the VA hospitals. Dr. Magnuson advocated carrying this plan one step further by having the hospitals affiliated with nearby medical schools.

Although previously indifferent to the VA's medical program, and in fact disapproving of its policy of providing care to veterans without regard to financial need or connection with war service, the AMA pledged its enthusiastic support of General Hawley's proposal. The timing was right; nothing was too good for the veterans four months after VJ Day.

Dr. Magnuson took leave from his practice and teaching responsibilities at Northwestern, joined General Hawley as acting assistant medical director for research and education, and the Hawley-Magnuson team went into action.* Having sold the scheme to the VA and the AMA they were now faced with the problem of convincing the medical schools of its validity. Within four months, 80 percent of the medical schools had agreed to cooperate. Considering the inertia usually associated with such ventures, the speed with which their objective was achieved is amazing. It is equally amazing that the union of these state and private institutions and the federal government took place with so little formality: there were no

---

* Dr. Magnuson succeeded General Hawley as chief medical director in 1948.

written contracts, legal clauses, or memoranda of intent or agreement—merely an exchange of letters.

Basic to the plan was the concept that it would have two objectives: elevation of the quality of medical care in the VA hospitals, and the specialty training of young physicians. The medical schools were informed that, upon acknowledgement of their willingness to cooperate, the VA hospital staffs would henceforth be appointed on recommendation of committees consisting of the deans and members of the medical school faculties. The committees were to be the sole judges of professional standards. There were to be "senior consultants" of professional rank responsible for the overall supervision and guidance of clinical services and teaching; "consultants" to be chosen at first from among board-certified physicians who had taught in medical schools prior to military service; and "ward officers" who would receive resident-type training. Positions as ward officers would be open primarily to younger discharged medical officers, and physicians on the VA rolls who desired specialty training and certification.

The expedient arrangements on which the affiliations had been based were strengthened by passage by Congress of P.L. 293 in 1946, which established the VA's Department of Medicine and Surgery and legitimized the Hawley-Magnuson organization. The bill provided that appointment of professional personnel would be made after their qualifications had been satisfactorily established in accordance with regulations, and without regard to civil service requirements. A most important provision, from the educational standpoint, was the authority it gave the VA to establish residencies, in place of ward officers, in affiliated teaching hospitals.

Following enactment of P.L. 293 the gentlemen's agreements between the central office of the VA and the medical schools were strengthened and defined by a statement known as "Policy Memorandum No. 2," which prescribed their respective responsibilities and those of the hospital managers, chiefs of service, and attending and consultant staffs. This remarkable document, brief and devoid of legal verbiage, was still in effect, with little modification, twenty-four years later.

There was no clause in either P.L. 293 or Policy Memorandum No. 2 that either permitted or prohibited use of the affiliated veterans hospitals for instruction at the predoctoral level. Nevertheless, the medical schools soon realized that in these hospitals, staffed by competent members of their faculties, was a wealth of teaching material not being utilized. Enrollment of medical students had increased during the war, and the distribution of patient populations in general hospitals was beginning to change as the length of stay decreased, and as more patients covered by insurance were admitted to private services. Assignment of clinical clerks to the veterans hospitals would not only provide contact with a larger number of patients but experience in dealing with long-term illness: patients with chronic pulmonary, neurological, orthopedic, and neuropsychiatric disorders were available in abundance. Within a few months, medical students were working in some veterans hospitals, and in 1948 an official bulletin sanctioned what had been going on for two years.

From the beginning, the extent of affiliation between the medical schools and the veterans hospitals differed widely. Some hospitals were located at great distance from a medical school, while others were devoted almost exclusively to domiciliary care; in these instances a meaningful relationship was difficult to work out. Other hospitals, located in urban centers where there were several medical schools, had multiple affiliations. These relationships were generally less satisfactory because "what is everyone's business is no one's business," and the degree of responsibility of each of the several schools was usually less than in cases where a one-to-one relationship prevailed.

By 1948, sixty-eight veterans hospitals were affiliated with fifty-eight medical schools. Over the next several years it became the policy of the federal government to build new hospitals in close proximity to medical schools whenever possible. Some of the isolated rural hospitals were closed, and some affiliations established early in the program were discontinued, usually due to lack of accessibility. By 1965 ninety veterans hospitals were affiliated with seventy-seven medical schools. They provided approximately 20 percent of all the hospital beds used for teaching in the United States.

The impact of the medical school–Veterans Administration relationship was not limited to the availability of teaching facilities for residents and medical students. It elevated the quality of medical service immeasurably, and probably saved the federal government a considerable amount of money by shortening the length of hospitalization and removing many veterans from the rolls of disabled pensioners. Medical education benefited by having faculty members' salaries and research laboratories financed by the federal government. All told, it was one of those mutually advantageous arrangements that result from having the right people involved at the right time. It would be difficult to attribute too much credit to the inspired leadership of General Hawley and Dr. Magnuson, and to the foresight of the medical profession in those crucial days at the end of World War II.

NOTE

1. This chapter is based largely on a report prepared by B. J. Lewis for the House of Representatives Committee on Veterans Affairs: *Veterans Administration Medical Program Relationship with Medical Schools in the United States* (Washington: U.S. Government Printing Office, House Committee Print No. 170, 91st Congress, 2nd session, 1970.)

VIII. The Impact of Research

A REVIEW of advances in medical science over the half century under consideration will not be attempted here; comments in this chapter will be limited to the impact of expanding research activity on the educational process and on the atmosphere of the medical schools.[1]

It would be difficult for one who has not lived through this period to appreciate the extent to which the introduction of research on a large scale changed the character of American medical schools. By 1920 the more progressive schools were becoming scientifically oriented, and small amounts of research support were being provided by foundations. Research activity was stimulated largely by personal initiative rather than by institutional pressures. Throughout the next twenty years a growing interest in research became evident, as did correspondingly increased rewards in prestige for those so engaged. The economic depression of the 1930s, however, forced the universities to reduce research activities in order to maintain essential instructional functions.

FEDERAL SUPPORT

Health research had become established as a social endeavor worthy of support, and this fact was recognized by the federal government. Legislation in 1930 changed the name of the Hygienic Laboratory, established in 1887, to the National Institute of Health and provided for its operation. The appropriation for its support in fiscal year 1931 was only $43,000, however, and it increased very slowly over the next decade. Although money was in short supply, there was a rise in national concern for the social and economic security of the people, reflected in the passage in 1937 of the National Cancer Act which created the National Cancer Institute and provided for grants-in-aid for nonfederal research projects and fellowships for advanced training of medical scientists.

With the beginning of World War II and the establishment of the Office of Scientific Research and Development (OSRD), the federal government's concern about the organization of medical research related to military problems led to appropriations far in excess of those available previously. Medical schools, as well as other divisions of the universities, suddenly became responsible for large-scale and well-financed research programs.

The end of World War II found biomedical sciences ready for a major expansion. A pool of professional manpower was prepared to develop this potential beyond the capacity of universities and foundations to support it. Wartime contracts under the OSRD were transferred to the National Institute of Health and the Office of Naval Research, and the federal government was committed to continue support of scientific endeavors beyond the walls of its own institutions.

With the founding of the National Science Foundation in 1950 the decision was made to assign major responsibility for federal support of research in the physical sciences to that agency, and in the biomedical sciences to the National Institute of Health. In the same year broad legislation known as the "PHS Omnibus Act" empowered the surgeon general to establish separate institutes to deal with major disease problems. Categorical institutes to be concerned with neurological diseases and blindness, arthritis and metabolic diseases, and allergy and infectious diseases were founded, and the National Institute of Health became the National Institutes of Health (NIH). Each institute was to conduct research in its field within the expanding NIH complex in Bethesda and also to administer grants-in-aid to nonfederal institutions. Much of the credit for this program is attributable to the foresight of Leonard A. Scheele, the surgeon general from 1948 to 1956, and to the fortunate selection of James A. Shannon as director of the NIH, a position he held from 1955 to 1969.

Another decision made at this time that had a far-reaching effect on relations between the federal government and the scientific community was the establishment of panels of experts, which became known as "study sections," to judge the scientific merits of research proposals. Judgment as to the quality and relevance of research projects was thus removed from the bureaucracy. This decision may account for the wise policy that fundamental biological research receive consideration equal to that which holds promise of immediate returns in diagnosis and therapy.

It soon became apparent that the research potential exceeded the availability of facilities. Although expansion of the NIH at Bethesda had provided for intramural research, little had been done to provide the space needed in the medical schools to carry out their share of the programs. School buildings that had been marginally adequate for instruction and the small-scale research projects of the prewar era were totally inadequate to meet the increased demands of expanding programs and personnel. It was said at the time that if people were not working in closets, and if apparatus were not placed in the corridors, the laboratories were not being properly utilized. Passage of the Health Research Facilities Construction Act of 1956 contributed substantially to overcoming this problem. Under this legislation, matching funds—50 percent of cost—were provided for the construction of and basic equipment for research facilities in nonfederal institutions, principally medical schools. The response to this stimulus was quite amazing, and, with the promise of federal funds as bait, sources of funds that had been most difficult to tap became available. State legislatures, individual donors, and even foundations that had persisted in maintaining a "no bricks and mortar" policy loosened their purse strings. Few medical schools failed to take advantage of the opportunity not only to expand and improve their research laboratories, but such supporting elements as animal quarters. This program remained in operation over the next dozen years but was curtailed and finally abolished during the Nixon administration.

It was realized in the 1950s that encouragement of the national research effort in medical science also required an investment in the training of personnel. Funds for pre- and postdoctoral research fellowships and training programs were therefore provided by the federal government in increased amounts. Career research professorships that guaranteed salaries until retirement were funded in limited numbers by the NIH, the American Cancer Society, and the American Heart Association.

General research support grants, distributed in proportion to the volume of research in progress at medical schools and other institutions, provided unrestricted funds for salaries of research personnel, equipment, and seed money for the initiation of new research projects. Expanded opportunities for clinical investigation were provided in teaching hospitals through support of units of beds termed "clinical research centers," where patients could remain for study, beyond the period necessary for their diagnosis or treatment, at no expense to themselves.

Without attempting a complicated analysis of the economics of the federal program, its growth can be illustrated by a quotation from a lecture by Dr. Shannon at the 1966 meeting of the AAMC:

> In 1947 the national expenditure for medical research totaled $87 million, of which the federal share was $27 million, or 31 percent. The National Institutes of Health that year expended $8.3 million, or 10 percent of the national effort. For 1966, the national medical research expenditures are estimated at $2.05 billion, exclusive of construction and training. The federal component is $1.4 billion, or 68 percent; and the NIH portion amounts to $800 million, or 40 percent of the whole. A signal fact of this twenty-year comparison is that total dollars available for the nation's medical research have increased twenty-four times. If the Gross National Product deflation factor is applied to correct for price and wage changes over this period, the increase is still in the order of fifteen times.[2]

A continued increase in medical research expenditures at the same pace could hardly have been expected, and funding began to plateau in 1967.

The figures quoted above do not include a breakdown that

shows the impact of federal support of medical research on the finances of the medical schools. The following quotation from an address by Thomas B. Turner at the same AAMC meeting clarifies this point:

> The total funds available to the NIH in fiscal 1966 for extramural support of research, including construction of research facilities, was approximately $1.2 billion. It is estimated that, overall, about 50 percent of these funds were granted to medical schools, with the remainder going to other components of the universities, to independent hospitals, and to non-university research organizations.[3]

In other words, in fiscal 1966 the medical schools then in operation received in the neighborhood of $600 million from the NIH.

Much of the credit for this enlightened attitude of the federal government may be attributed to the wisdom of Dr. Shannon, the farsighted leadership of Marion B. Folsom, secretary of health, education, and welfare during the Eisenhower administration, and to Senator Lister Hill and Congressman John E. Fogarty, who were deeply convinced of the validity of the health research program and steered appropriations through the Congress.

The Medical Schools Adjust

As scientific research became a dominant feature of the academic scene, medical schools and their parent universities had to make many difficult adjustments. The stability and balance of interests in the schools were seriously threatened. Departmental interests often became centered on one or two superior and well-supported research programs, and departments that were successful in obtaining large grants overshadowed their less aggressive colleagues in the competition for space and budgetary allocations. Better management and accounting procedures as well as supporting services had to be established.

Long-term planning became difficult as sources of support

became less predictable. In 1968–69 approximately one-third of faculty salaries were paid from federal sources, and 58 percent of the total budgets of all medical schools were derived from outside sources.

The average faculty member had to adapt to a new way of life. Instead of working in the laboratory as an individual, he became the manager of a research team consisting of more junior faculty members, postdoctoral fellows, technicians, and secretaries. Skill in composing research proposals often determined his recognition and advancement. He was on a treadmill, constantly concerned over his current grant, and over the preparation of an equally inspired application for renewal when it expired. His loyalty to the school tended to diminish as he became dependent on outside sources for support of his research, and often for at least a portion of his salary. If local conditions were not to his liking he could pack up and move to another institution, taking his support and auxiliary personnel with him. Loss of security on the part of investigators was often damaging to the morale of the institution.

The impact of the federal medical research program on the educational programs of the medical schools was generally favorable. It has been said that it diverted the schools from their primary mission of developing practicing physicians, but there is no data to support this contention. On the contrary, during the period the program was in operation there was a substantial rise in the number of graduates. The proportional increase in full-time faculty members was far greater, with resultant availability of teachers with specialized knowledge and skills in a wider variety of subdisciplines. Although the absolute number of graduates entering careers in teaching and research expanded, the proportion was not great.[4] Only 2.7 percent of interns in 1964–65 indicated research or teaching, without clinical responsibilities, as their career choice.

One of the interesting developments over this fifty-year period was the change in the research interests of medical faculty members. Early in this period clinicians made clinical observations on patients, and, if they worked in the laboratory, they examined human blood, excreta, exudates, and tissues.

Training for a year or two in a pathology laboratory was considered a highly desirable experience for a young physician looking forward to a career in academic medicine. Even basic scientists who were members of medical faculties tended to work on problems of immediate relevance to clinical medicine. Over the years, more and more young clinicians went to work in physiological, biochemical, and microbiological laboratories and became highly proficient in some aspect of one of these disciplines. Many laboratories in clinical departments became oriented to basic research and animal experimentation. Simultaneously, the basic medical scientists transferred their interests to the cellular and subcellular levels and had more difficulty in communicating with their clinical colleagues. Clinical teachers became capable of explaining symptoms and the rationale of therapy on the basis of the alterations of physiological processes that characterized diseases. Students obtained a better understanding of biological science as a foundation for clinical medicine, although they tended to be impatient with instruction that seemed remote from medical practice.

It seems probable that medical scientists of the future, including clinical investigators, will consider a foundation in one of the basic sciences essential. Toward the end of this period, graduates holding both M.D. and Ph.D. degrees were being produced in increasing numbers and were being appointed in both clinical and basic science departments.

The creation of a considerate, understanding physician, sensitive to the problems and needs of his patients, their families, and society as a whole, is certainly a desirable objective of medical education; the creation of a scholarly, scientific physician is equally important. He must have the ability to acquire, evaluate, store, and integrate available information; he must know how to produce and evaluate new data and to solve new clinical problems; and he must deal with drugs that are potentially extremely dangerous if not used wisely and cautiously. That physicians trained in an atmosphere of scientific research are more likely to acquire these capabilities is hard to deny; that compassion and a scientific atitude are incompatible is a contention equally difficult to support.

The invasion of the research establishment over these fifty years had a highly desirable influence on American medical education. In retrospect it is fortunate that the United States did not follow the policy adopted by other nations of segregating medical research in institutes that were independent of or only loosely connected with universities.

NOTES

1. For further information on this subject, see: J. H. Comroe, ed., "Research and Medical Education," *Journal of Medical Education* 37 (1962); *Reform of Medical Education: The Role of Research in Medical Education* (Washington: U.S. Government Printing Office, 1970); and G. H. Rosen, "Patterns of Health Research in the United States, 1900–1960," *Bulletin of the History of Medicine* 39 (1965): 201.

2. J. A. Shannon, "The Advancement of Medical Research: A Twenty-Year View of the Role of the National Institutes of Health," *Journal of Medical Education* 42 (1967): 97.

3. T. B. Turner, "The Medical Schools Twenty Years Afterwards: Impact of the Extramural Research Support Programs of the National Institutes of Health," *Journal of Medical Education* 42 (1967): 109.

4. P. J. Sanazaro, "Class Size in Medical School," *Journal of Medical Education* 41 (1966): 1017.

IX. Licensure

IN many countries completion of a standardized educational program in medicine and award of a degree or certificate automatically convey the right to practice. In the United States, however, education and licensure have remained separate but related, and only this relationship will be discussed here. Excellent monographs on the history of licensure, including extensive bibliographies, are available.[1]

In the period prior to 1820, when few practicing physicians had any formal education, efforts were made to establish a system of licensure. Contradictory as it may seem, the founding of medical colleges and the prestige accorded to them encouraged deterioration of the licensing procedure. Degrees became accepted as superior to licenses, and were sought by most individuals entering the profession. To meet the demand for diplomas, proprietary medical schools of dubious quality proliferated and the situation was completely out-of-hand throughout most of the nineteenth century.

States rights were so firmly supported that no system of national licensure was feasible, and attempts to regulate the profession at the state level ran contrary to the spirit of individualism and anti-intellectualism associated with Jacksonian democracy. There was controversy as to whether control should be the responsibility of the states, the profession, or the schools. The issue was further complicated by the appearance of homeopaths, eclectics, and other sects that divided the profession.

A compromise was found in the establishment of state boards of medical examiners composed of physicians, officially or unofficially nominated by the state medical societies, whose functions were regulated by state governments. Cumulative efforts to integrate the independent boards and encourage reciprocity led the state examiners to organize, and in 1891 the National Confederation of State Medical and Licensing Boards, later to become the Federation of State Medical Boards (FSMB), was founded.

This system of state licensure had many defects. It inhibited mobility at a time when new frontiers were opening in the West; and the volume and diversity of regulations, and strict interpretation of many legal requirements, led to rigidity and the overcrowding of the curriculum and discouraged innovative practices. One of the first actions of the Commission on Medical Education,[2]* organized in 1925, was a recommendation to the FSMB that a truce be established during which any member school of the AAMC might experiment with medical education without penalty to its graduates. A revision of the constitution and by-laws of the federation, adopted in 1930, contained the following provision:

> In all matters of premedical education, courses of study, and educational requirements for the degree of Doctor of Medicine or its equivalent, the Federation recognizes the Association of American Medical Colleges as the standardizing agency for this purpose. The Federation regards as its proper function (a) the determining of fitness for the practice of medicine, and (b) the enforcement of regulatory measures.[3]

National Board of Medical Examiners

National licensure along the lines adopted by other countries seemed unattainable, even though uniform standards and improved opportunity for mobility were highly desirable. The establishment in 1915 of a voluntary agency, the National Board of Medical Examiners (NBME), provided such a solution. While power to license was retained by the forty-eight state boards, they could accept the certificate of examination issued by the NBME in lieu of their own examinations.

Indirectly, the NBME influenced the quality of medical

* For a description of how the commission was organized, see Chapter XI, page 101.

education because it set requirements for admission to its examinations that were higher than those of most of the states. Requirements included a diploma from a four-year high school; a satisfactory college course in the natural sciences; graduation from a Grade A medical school; and at least one year's internship in an acceptable hospital. The limitation of applicants to graduates of Grade A schools was particularly important because it reinforced the recommendations of the Flexner Report and exerted further pressure on schools to secure an A rating.

The NBME also introduced a professional approach to examination for licensure that had been lacking in the state examinations. Instead of the oral presentations and case demonstrations, it developed a three-part program: Part I was a written examination in the basic medical sciences; Part II a written examination in clinical medicine; and Part III a practical examination at the bedside. Eligibility to take each examination was dependent on successful completion of the previous one. Part I was usually taken after the second year in medical school, Part II at the end of the fourth year, and Part III after internship. Prior to 1950, Parts I and II were essay-type examinations; thereafter, multiple-choice tests were substituted.

As the expertise of the NBME became recognized, it was called upon to assist other organizations in the development of their examining procedures. A multiple-choice examination known as FLEX was made available to the state boards of medical examiners and widely substituted for the oral and essay tests that had been used previously. With the aid of the NBME, many of the specialty boards developed multiple-choice examinations adapted to their requirements; professional associations requested assistance in development of self-assessment tests; and for internal examinations medical schools used "minitests" composed of selected NBME questions.

The NBME examinations, designed originally to evaluate the *product* of medical education, became in time an instrument for evaluation of the *process*. The performances of students in a given discipline at one school could be compared with those of students at other schools, and instructional weaknesses could thus be detected and corrected.[4]

The extensive revisions of the medical curriculum that were introduced in the late 1960s (see Chapter II) led to reconsideration of the NBME examination schedule and brought up the question as to when a license for independent practice should be granted. Since the new curriculum had eliminated the sharp division between preclinical and clinical studies, separate Parts I and II examinations were no longer realistic. There was need for a single examination at the time of graduation that would determine whether the candidate had sufficient knowledge of the fundamentals of medical science and technology to justify his entering upon a phase of training in which he would master the skills necessary for the competent practice of his specialty. Part III was about to become equally unrealistic because the internship year was destined to be eliminated.

At the 1968 meeting of the NBME a proposal was made to combine Parts I and II in a single examination to be taken upon graduation: it would be known as the Qualifying Examination, Part A. On passing it the recent graduate would be issued a provisional license permitting him to practice under supervision in an institution. The specialty board examination, to be known as the Qualifying Examination, Part B, would be taken on completion of residency training and would test for competence in a special field of medicine or surgery. This would lead to full licensure and the right to practice independently. The proposal also noted that permanent licensure disregards the fact that people and medical knowledge change, and that the system should include provision for periodic reexamination.[5] Five years later a committee appointed to study this proposal recommended its acceptance [6] and it was taken under further consideration by the NBME and other organizations.

A legal basis for medical licensure had been established in all the states by 1920, and it was altered very little over the following fifty years. A detailed analysis of the individual laws and regulations is beyond the scope of this book, but, in general, to be eligible for licensure an American physician had to be a graduate of an "approved" medical school, pass either state or NBME examinations, and serve a one-year internship in an "approved" hospital. Most state laws required that approval of the schools be the responsibility of either the AAMC or the AMA, or both. In actual practice, inspection and approval of the schools were carried out cooperatively by the Liaison Committee on Medical Education of the two associations, and their endorsements coincided.

Foreign Medical Graduates

Throughout these fifty years the licensing of graduates of foreign medical schools presented a special problem.[7] Americans who were unable to gain admission to schools at home obtained diplomas from European schools, and with the rise of fascism in the 1930s a large number of Central European physicians migrated to the United States.* The state of New York, where the pressure was greatest, attempted to establish a list of acceptable foreign schools, but this was a futile endeavor and, in general, candidates were admitted to examinations on an individual basis, usually after serving internships in American hospitals.

A second wave of foreign graduates attracted to the United States after World War II consisted largely of non-European physicians, many of whom not only had an inferior medical education but language difficulties.† Available hospital internships far exceeded the number of graduates of American schools, so foreign graduates had little difficulty in obtaining temporary employment. To deal with this problem a committee representing the FSMB, the AAMC, the American

---

* Physicians examined for licensure on the basis of credentials obtained in countries other than the United States and Canada soared from 437 in 1935 to 2,088 in 1940. By 1970 the number had reached 6.236, equivalent to 74 percent of United States graduates in that year.

† Sixty-six percent of physicians admitted to the United States as immigrants in 1971 were from Asia, principally from India, the Philippines, and Korea.

Hospital Association, and the AMA Council on Medical Education was appointed in 1954 to devise "an effective mechanism for measuring educational attainment in the absence of intimate knowledge of the educational background of foreign physicians." This led to the establishment in 1957 of the Educational Council for Foreign Medical Graduates (ECFMG). Examinations in English as well as in the basic sciences and clinical medicine were held at centers in the United States and abroad, with the cooperation of American embassies.* Theoretically, only those who passed the ECFMG examination could be appointed to internships or sit for state board examinations, but the former restriction was not rigidly enforced.

The idea behind establishing the ECFMG was sound. It was assumed that a modest number of foreign graduates would be coming to the United States for advanced training, that they would return to their native countries, and that few would seek licensure. They were classified as exchange visitors and students rather than as immigrants. The examination was designed to determine the likelihood of their profiting from the learning experience, and whether or not they had the clinical competence to be trusted with the limited responsibilities of an intern.

In reality, the number of foreign graduates who passed the ECFMG and entered the United States with the intention of obtaining licenses and residing here permanently increased annually. They could no longer be considered exchange students but, rather, prospective members of the medical profession in this country. At the same time, the United States became concerned about a shortage of physicians, and the national immigration policy encouraged entry of any individual recognized as a doctor in his native country, regardless of his qualifications.

As the number of foreign medical graduates licensed each

---

* The number taking the ECFMG examinations increased annually: in 1970, 29,950 took the examinations, and 39.8 percent passed.

year approached the number graduating from American schools, public concern grew. Licensure had for years been based on the concept that the applicant was both adequately educated and able to pass an examination. Foreign graduates were being licensed on the basis of repeated, and finally successful, efforts to first pass the ECFMG and then state board examinations, with little regard to the quality of their education.

In summary, while some progress in the regulation of the practice of medicine was made over this fifty-year period, the ultimate goal of a national system of licensure and registration had not been attained. Perhaps that is just as well. National licensure administered by a bureaucracy entails the danger of stultifying control of curriculum and standards. Conscientious self-regulation of the educational program by the medical profession and academic establishment has the advantage of avoiding inhibition of innovative practices that are responsive to advances in medical science as well as to changing social conditions.

NOTES

1. See: R. H. Shryock, *Medical Licensing in America, 1650–1965* (Baltimore: Johns Hopkins Press, 1967); and R. C. Derbyshire, *Medical Licensure and Discipline in the United States* (Baltimore: Johns Hopkins Press, 1969).

2. Commission on Medical Education, *Final Report of the Commission on Medical Education* (New York: Office of the Director of the Study, 1932).

3. W. C. Rappleye, "Major Changes in Medical Education During the Past Fifty Years," *Journal of Medical Education* 34 (1959): 683.

4. J. P. Hubbard, *Measuring Medical Education* (Philadelphia: Lea and Feibiger, 1971).

5. V. W. Lippard, "How Should the National Board Respond to Changing Patterns of Medical Education?" *The National Board Examiner* 15, no. 7 (1968).

6. *Evaluation of the Continuum of Medical Education* (Philadelphia: National Board of Medical Examiners, 1973).

7. For detailed consideration of the problems of licensing foreign graduates, see: J. Z. Bowers and Lord Rosenheim, *Migration of Medical Manpower* (New York: Josiah Macy, Jr. Foundation, 1971); H. Margulies and L. S. Bloch, *Foreign Medical Graduates in the United States* (Cambridge: Harvard University Press, 1969); and R. Stevens and J. Vermeulen, *Foreign Trained Physicians and American Medicine* (Washington: Division of Manpower Intelligence, Division of Health Manpower Education, National Institutes of Health, DHEW Publication No. NIH 73-325, 1972).

X. Specialization and
the Specialty Boards

ONE of the most significant factors in altering the character of medical education and practice over the past fifty years has been the increase in specialization.[1] During most of the nineteenth century, medical practice had been an individual endeavor with little control or institutionalization; medical education followed the same pattern. Toward the end of the century, however, the population became more urban; hospitals were organized; and the tendency of physicians to emphasize one aspect of medical practice, rather than limit it to a specialty, became more apparent.

Because of a dearth of formal training programs leading to specialization, most of those who became recognized as specialists by their colleagues, and consequently were called upon as consultants, attained that status by independent study and apprenticeship. The alternate route was didactic instruction at one of the postgraduate medical schools that flourished in this country and in Europe. The most popular schools in the United States were in New York, Philadelphia, and Chicago, and abroad in Vienna and Berlin. The courses lasted for a few weeks to a year, consisted of lectures and demonstrations, and seldom involved any practical experience.

By 1920 the division of teaching hospital services by specialty, and the consequent similar organization of medical faculties, was well established. The first separation of surgeons and general practitioners came with the development of anesthesia and aseptic surgery. The development of equipment and surgical skills was leading to subspecialization in surgery, but even in the leading university hospitals it was still not uncommon for the general surgeon to do a thoracotomy one day and remove a brain tumor the next. The major specialties of internal medicine, obstetrics and gynecology, pediatrics, and psychiatry became recognized later. Nevertheless, approximately 80 percent of practitioners were still listed as generalists, and outside the hospitals there was little regulation.

Protection of society from the untrained and unskilled physician with an urge to operate required some form of control, and debate ensued as to the advisability of accomplishing this by licensure or by the formation of guilds. The latter approach seemed more feasible, and the American College of Surgeons (ACS) was founded in 1913 under the leadership of the most prestigious surgeons of the day. Organization of the American College of Physicians followed two years later.

Development of the Boards

At about the same time, doctors who had become highly skilled in refraction and the treatment of diseases of the eye resented the competition of "six-week specialists" and opticians who did not hold medical degrees. In an effort to recognize competence in this field the ophthalmologists adopted a different approach. The three organizations concerned were the AMA Section of Ophthalmology, the American Ophthalmological Society, and the American Academy of Ophthalmology and Otolaryngology. Instead of founding a new association, as did the surgeons, the three societies joined in 1916 to form the American Board for Ophthalmic Examinations (ABOE), renamed the American Board of Ophthalmology in 1933. Its chief functions were to establish standards of competence to practice the specialty; to conduct examinations that would test qualifications; and to confer certificates. Older men with recognized competence were granted certificates under a "grandfather clause"; others were required to have two years of graduate study and one year of supervised clinical experience in order to qualify for examination. Thus the ABOE became both a prescriber of training standards and an examining body. Furthermore, the sponsoring societies agreed to limit membership to those who had been certified. Despite lack of any legal authority it became a potent force in the regulation of specialty practice and graduate education, and established a pattern that was to be followed by the other specialties.

Although self-declared eye, ear, nose, and throat specialists prospered before the ABOE was established, that event prophesied a division into two groups, the ophthalmologists and the otolaryngologists, and in 1924 the latter set up a separate American Board of Otolaryngology.

Spurred on by the maternal and child health movement, which had social and philanthropic as well as professional origins, the American Board of Obstetrics and Gynecology and the American Board of Pediatrics were founded in 1930 and 1932 under the sponsorship of their respective professional societies. By the end of that decade there were fifteen specialty boards; by 1970 there were twenty.

The establishment of boards in general surgery and the surgical specialties was more controversial than it had been in other fields. Membership in the American College of Surgeons, which antedated the board movement, was originally considered to be the badge of competence for all surgeons. The standards for admission were, however, lower than those for the boards, consisting of one year of internship, two years of surgical apprenticeship, and the presentation of case reports, but no formal examination. Furthermore, some of the surgical specialties were beginning to declare their independence. The American boards of orthopedic surgery, colon and rectal surgery, and anesthesiology were established between 1934 and 1936. Under pressure from academic surgeons who were represented in both the ACS and the prestigious American Surgical Association, the American Board of Surgery was finally established in 1937.

THE GENERAL PRACTITIONER

In retrospect it seems quite remarkable that this system of boards and board certification worked out as well as it did. From the very beginning it tended to downgrade the general practitioner as the man who was left over, who had no special competence, and who was therefore second-rate. The blame for this cannot be attributed entirely to the specialist groups. The Academy of General Practice,* founded in 1947, held that a general practitioner was a physician who did not specialize, with the implication that he was therefore qualified to do anything he chose. This was without doubt unwise strategically because, as the specialties carved out their territories, it left the general practitioner without a definite area of competence.

If the United States had followed the lead of Great Britain in the 1940s and established a national program for payment of health services, the decline of the generalist might have been forestalled. Defeat of the Murray-Wagner-Dingell bill,† however, put an end to movements in that direction until the Medicare and Medicaid programs were legislated in 1965. A concerted effort by the leaders of academic medicine might have turned the tide, and although a few socially conscious liberals among them supported the legislation vigorously, most of them were too busy to assume active roles. This was a period in which medical faculties were being reorganized and expanded to meet the challenges of rapidly developing research programs and their concerns were in other directions.

Throughout the period during which specialization was expanding, there was beneath the surface an awareness of the

---

* The Academy of General Practice later became the Academy of Family Practice and was instrumental in establishing the American Board of Family Practice.

† Agitation for national health insurance was brought to a climax with the introduction to Congress of the National Health Act of 1945, sponsored by Senators Murray and Wagner and Congressman Dingell. It provided for comprehensive, compulsory health insurance, to be financed by a 3 percent payroll tax on wages up to $3,600 a year. The bill was opposed vigorously by organized medicine and was never enacted.

need to perpetuate a corps of physicians who would establish a stable and continuing relationship with their patients and serve as general managers and coordinators of their health care. There was little in the educational system, however, that tended to encourage such a movement. Medical school curricula and internship programs were designed to turn out undifferentiated physicians, and those who dropped out on completion of the internship became general practitioners. This concept was reinforced by the Commission on Graduate Medical Education,[2] which maintained that the internships of those who planned to enter general practice and those who were to enter residency training and become specialists should be the same.

From time to time there were proposals that the role of the generalist be defined and his status improved by the establishment of a specialty board, but this movement was slow in gaining momentum. The founding of the Academy of General Practice may have postponed action because it provided a guild with which the generalist could be identified. Definitive action followed the report in 1966 of the Citizens Commission on Graduate Medical Education, a group sponsored by the AMA and chaired by John S. Millis, which endorsed board certification of primary or family practitioners.[3]

The first examinations of the American Board of Family Practice were held in 1970. The policies of this board included two radical innovations: there would be no grandfather clause, and periodic recertification would be required.

COORDINATION OF THE BOARDS

By 1933 five self-perpetuating specialty boards were in operation, and it was evident that this system would probably advance rapidly. The final report of the Commission on Medical Education * had recently been published,[4] and al-

---

* For a description of how the commission was organized, see Chapter XI, page 101.

though it dealt primarily with undergraduate medical education, members of the commission were concerned about the period of training that followed award of the M.D. degree. The boards had been formed by professional associations and lacked the coordination that would assure the maintenance of standards or prevent unwise fragmentation of the profession. Their standards differed, and they had no formal association with the universities. At the meeting of the Congress on Medical Education and Hospitals in February 1933 an informal group that represented the power structure met to consider this problem.* An outgrowth of this meeting was the formal organization of the Advisory Board for Medical Specialties a year later.

The advisory board was composed originally of representatives of the existing specialty boards, the AAMC, the NBME, the FSMB, and several other medical organizations. The Council on Medical Education of the AMA declined to accept membership on the grounds that it claimed final authority to regulate the boards, and that the advisory board should report to it. Despite this struggle for dominance, cooperative arrangements were made and common policies adopted. The "Essentials for an Approved Specialty Examining Board" were endorsed in virtually identical form, and new boards were established with joint sanction of the advisory board and the AMA.

With the publication of the first *Directory of Medical Specialists* in 1940,[5] those who were certified were clearly identified and separated from those who were not, thus further downgrading the status of the general practitioner. World War II served to strengthen the division because those who were certified or well along in their residencies were usually

---

* The leading figures were Willard C. Rappleye, formerly director of the study of the Commission on Medical Education, and then dean of the Columbia University College of Physicians and Surgeons; William Cutter, secretary of the Council on Medical Education of the AMA; Walter Bierring, an influential member of the American College of Physicians and of the Federation of State Medical Boards; Louis B. Wilson of the Mayo Clinic; Ray Lyman Wilbur, president of Stanford University; and Robin Buerki, spokesman for the American Hospital Association.

given the preferred assignments in military hospitals, while the less-trained manned induction stations or became battalion surgeons.

The growth of specialization and specialty boards affected medical education in many subtle ways. Certification became a requirement for appointment to many hospital staffs, particularly on the surgical services. Although universities denied that faculty appointments could be determined by outside professional organizations, they were influenced indirectly because of the importance of hospital staff privileges. The AMA established the requirements for and, after inspection, approved internships; and it joined with the specialty boards in approving residencies and determining the training requirements for board examinations. Thus an important phase of medical education passed out of the control of the medical schools and universities.

At the end of the period with which this book is concerned, and after thirty-seven years of indeterminate status, the Advisory Board for Medical Specialties was reorganized and its position strengthened; after 1970 it was to be known as the American Board of Medical Specialties. It would continue to consider approval of new specialty boards as they arose, through a liaison committee that included AMA representation; issue the *Directory of Medical Specialists;* provide a forum for discussion among board members; and have authority to generate educational and manpower studies.

Failure to Control the Production of Specialists

Despite this progress toward rational regulation of specialty board proliferation and adoption of common standards, many problems related to specialty education and practice fell between the authority or interests of the several organizations. Among them was the question of numerical production. The AMA Council on Medical Education imposed no controls over the number of residencies available in the various specialties or the number of hospitals approved as training centers. The council viewed its role as one of accreditation, and it was prepared to approve all hospitals that met minimal educational standards. Resident positions available in the hospitals reflected their need for personnel to meet service requirements: in time the availability of such positions exceeded the number of graduates of American schools who could fill them,* and many of the posts were occupied by foreign graduates.† As a result there was no relationship between supply and demand for specialists in the several fields. While family physicians and radiologists appeared to be in short supply, more than the necessary number of general surgeons were available, and excessive numbers were being trained in all of the surgical specialties.

Under the unorganized system that prevailed in 1970, only the roughest prediction of requirements was possible, and even if the figure were more accurate there was no way to enforce a better distribution. Three basic approaches were proposed. One was through a coordinated system of program accreditation in which the number and types of training centers and their enrollments would be redistributed in accordance with estimated needs; a second, probably impractical, proposal was dependent on regulating the supply of specialists in various fields by means of specialty board examinations; a third involved reorganization of residency training as an educational rather than an apprenticeship process, and university acceptance of responsibility for programs in regional affiliated hospitals. Under the third plan, a national commission would determine quotas in each of the specialties for each of the university-centered complexes, and perhaps guide the distribution of federal subsidies based on approved enrollments.

It appeared in 1970 that an adjustment in the rate of production and distribution of specialists, including the new specialty of family practice, was imperative from the stand-

---

* Between 1940 and 1970 the number of resident positions offered increased from 5,796 to 46,250; in the post–World War II period, approximately 80 percent of these positions were filled.

† In 1969, 32 percent of the interns and residents in United States hospitals were graduates of foreign medical schools.

points of both the medical profession and the public. How it could be accomplished outside the framework of a national health system, such as the one that had been so successful in Great Britain, was difficult to visualize.

NOTES

1. R. Stevens, *American Medicine and the Public Interest* (New Haven: Yale University Press, 1971). (The growth of specialization is treated exhaustively and an extensive bibliography on the subject is included.)

2. Commission on Graduate Medical Education, *Graduate Medical Education: Report of the Commission on Graduate Medical Education* (Chicago: University of Chicago Press, 1940).

3. Citizens Commission on Graduate Medical Education, *The Graduate Education of Physicians: Report of the Citizens Commission on Graduate Medical Education* (Chicago: American Medical Association, 1966).

4. Commission on Medical Education, *Final Report of the Commission on Medical Education* (New York: Office of the Director of Study, 1932).

5. *Directory of Medical Specialists* (Chicago: Marquis–Who's Who, Inc., published periodically since 1940).

XI. National Organizations and Foundations

ALMOST all of the events or trends mentioned in this book were influenced by one or more of the national organizations and foundations concerned primarily with medicine, education, or science. An adequate review of their activities over this half century would, however, require a volume of its own. Fortunately, the histories of several of these organizations are available.[1] Only a few of those whose impact on medical education appears to be most direct will be discussed here.

ASSOCIATION OF AMERICAN MEDICAL COLLEGES

At the top of the list is the Association of American Medical Colleges (AAMC). Founded in 1890, it provided a forum for discussions of medical education and, as the principal organization representing academic interests, balanced the more pragmatic and often economic and political concerns of the American Medical Association (AMA). During the first sixty years of its existence the AAMC functioned primarily as a "dean's club." With rare exceptions its officers were medical school deans who constituted the majority of those in attendance at its annual meetings.* The headquarters of the AAMC were in a downtown office building in Chicago, and the staff consisted of an executive secretary and a few clerks. It was

---

* The first AAMC meeting I attended was in 1939. It was held at the University of Michigan, where the group, totaling no more than one hundred, met in a classroom, and all were invited to a cocktail party at the dean's home. The 1970 meeting was held at the Biltmore Hotel in Los Angeles and had a registered attendance of over twenty-five hundred.

responsible for administering the Medical Aptitude Test, published the *Journal of the Association of American Medical Colleges* (later the *Journal of Medical Education*), and cooperated with the AMA in the inspection and accreditation of medical schools. While this accrediting body—the Liaison Committee on Medical Education—had no independent legal status, it had considerable power because eligibility for licensure in most states required graduation from an "approved medical school." The AAMC became much more active during the post–World War II decade as it assumed responsibility for the Medical College Admissions Test (1947) and the National Intern Matching Program (1952).

Having outgrown its office space in Chicago, and desirous of avoiding the high rent, the AAMC acquired land adjacent to Northwestern University in Evanston, Illinois, and, with the aid of a generous grant from the China Medical Board, constructed a building there which it occupied in late 1956.* This move coincided with the appointment of Ward Darley as executive director (1957) and the transition of the association from a rather bland and congenial organization, devoted largely to cordial exchanges of ideas and condolences, to a source of political influence in science and health. Dr. Darley, formerly dean of the medical school and later president of the University of Colorado, had been active in the AAMC for some years, having held the office of president in 1952–53. He had the background, wisdom, and energy that were so sorely needed at a time when the Congress and a substantial portion of the public had lost faith in the AMA, which was considered by many to be too concerned with the economics of medicine and preservation of the status quo. Under Dr. Darley's effective leadership the AAMC grew in power and influence over the next decade, a period in which federal support of medical research and education played such an important role in changing the character of American medical schools.

---

* It was discovered that although the AAMC had been in existence for sixty-five years it could not own property because it had never been incorporated. I was president of the AAMC at that time and consequently became the incorporator.

The next major step in the expansion and extension of the activities of the AAMC occurred in 1965 with the publication of the report, *Planning for Medical Progress through Education,* better known as the "Coggeshall Report." [2] Lowell T. Coggeshall, then vice president of the University of Chicago and formerly dean of its Division of Biological Sciences, as chairman of the AAMC committee that wrote the report, made a critical analysis of the organization, functions, and policies of the AAMC and established a plan for its evolution. The sixty recommendations in his report dealt with the AAMC's philosophy and objectives; programs; organization; membership; committee structure; relationships with other organizations and institutions; facilities; and financing. One of the immediate results was the transfer of the AAMC headquarters from Evanston to Washington, D.C., indicative of the expanded role it was to take in national affairs and in its relation to the federal government. At the same time a full-time executive was designated as president, the chief elected officer becoming chairman. The first full-time president was John A. D. Cooper, formerly vice president for science at Northwestern University.

Another significant development was the establishment of the Council of Teaching Hospitals as a division of the AAMC. Medical school deans and the directors of their closely affiliated hospitals were constantly aware of their interdependence at a local level, but had no established liaison at the national level. Whereas the American Hospital Association was concerned with hospital economics and management, the teaching hospitals were concerned also with education. The presence of hospital directors at the meetings of the council, and their participation with the deans in committee work, provided a common ground for the advancement of clinical instruction and research. Although at home they might continue to squabble over the division of the costs of educating students, interns, and residents, and the allocation of space, they found it advantageous to present a common front in dealing with outsiders, particularly the federal government.

In order to encourage the active participation of entire

faculties, rather than just their administrative officers, the AAMC organized the Council of Academic Societies, parallel to the Council of Teaching Hospitals. Fundamental and more meaningful than these organizational changes was the adoption of the concept that "the association should make it plain that it regards its role as one of serving the nation and public interest through institutions that compose it." Furthermore, the AAMC was to recognize even more clearly that medical education is a continuum and that its interests should extend beyond the predoctoral period to include postdoctoral and continuing education of health personnel. It also recommended that:

> . . . the professional aspects of education for health and medical sciences should be regarded as an essential function and a fully integrated component of university organization, with decreasing dependence upon or control by organized professions and their related associations.*

Two surveys of medical education, sponsored initially by the AAMC but financed to a large extent by foundations, deserve special mention.

The Commission on Medical Education, an influential group representing medical schools, universities, the profession, and licensing bodies, was established in 1925 and over the next several years conducted a comprehensive study of the whole field.† The final report of the commission, published in 1932, was written by Willard C. Rappleye, who subsequently served as dean of the College of Physicians and Surgeons of Columbia University for twenty-seven years.[3] The Flexner Report had gotten undergraduate medical education on the right track; this study marked the beginning of surveys on the relation of

---

* This recommendation was accepted less than warmly by some of the professional associations. The American College of Surgeons at its annual meeting on October 18, 1965, for example, resolved that: "The College shall indicate its disapproval of the plan outlined in the report by which the activities of the AAMC would be expanded widely to pre-empt the fields of postgraduate education, training and medical services."

† The impact of this study on licensure is discussed in Chapter IX, page 82; its concern with postgraduate training is discussed in Chapter X, pages 93–94.

the physician manpower supply to the demands and needs for service. Doctors were beginning to move from rural to urban areas, to become closely associated with hospitals, and to specialize, and the threat of maldistribution was becoming apparent. Attempts to solve these problems were still being made forty years later.

The next committee to make a major study of medical education, sponsored primarily by the AAMC and directed by John E. Dietrich and Robert C. Berson, published its report in 1953.[4] The rapid development of the fundamental sciences and their application to diagnosis and treatment had changed the character of medical schools, which were becoming large and highly complex institutions with research components that were inconceivable a few years earlier. In this report more attention was given to administration, finances, faculty organization, facilities, hospital relationships, residency training, research, and service than had seemed necessary in earlier studies. Medical schools were no longer the comfortable places they used to be; new opportunities and responsibilities were making management more complicated and the lives of faculty members and administrators less serene.

In 1951 and 1952 the AAMC cooperated with the American Psychiatric Association in the organization of two conferences on psychiatric education.[5] These conferences were significant for two reasons: first, they formulated a program of instruction designed to prepare the medical student to deal intelligently and skilfully with patients as persons, and to provide him with basic knowledge of psychological and social problems and resources in relation to health and disease; second, they set the pattern for a series of institutes, held over the following fifteen years, that dealt with instruction in the several biomedical disciplines and with such issues as medical school administration and teaching hospital relationships. The reports of these institutes, published as supplements to the *Journal of Medical Education,* provide an insight into the problems about which medical educators were concerned during the two decades after World War II.[6]

AMERICAN MEDICAL ASSOCIATION

The AMA was another organization that exerted a continuing influence on medical education, sometimes constructive and sometimes inhibiting. From its inception in 1847 the AMA had demonstrated its interest in elevating educational standards and in the need for a comprehensive investigation of the status of medical education, which led to the establishment in 1904 of the Council on Medical Education, later designated the Council on Medical Education and Hospitals.*

Although the AMA continued to have a declared interest in predoctoral education, often discussed it at its annual Conference on Medical Education and Licensure, published very valuable summaries of statistics and recent events in the annual educational numbers of the *Journal of the American Medical Association,* and continued to cooperate with the AAMC in the inspection of medical schools, its last serious and independent foray into that field was published in the report, *Medical Education in the United States, 1934–1939.*[7]

The addition of "hospitals" to the title of the council may have been indicative of its transfer of emphasis to education at the postdoctoral level. As internships and residencies became phases of medical education equal in importance to the predoctoral years, the AMA assumed entire responsibility for the inspection and approval of internships and, with the cooperation of the specialty boards, of residencies.

Characteristic of the AMA's interest in postdoctoral education was its sponsorship of the Citizens Commission on Graduate Medical Education. The commission took a hard look at the existing situation and recognized the gap between knowledge and practice; the rigid fragmentation of the several phases of medical education; the failure of many physicians to continue their education after termination of formal training; and the shortage of primary physicians. In its 1966 report the

---

* The council's participation in the study that led to the Flexner Report is discussed in Chapter I, page 3.

commission made a number of concrete recommendations, most significant of which were the following:

> We therefore recommend that graduation from medical school be recognized as the end of general medical education, and that specialized training begin with the start of graduate medical education. We recommend that the internship, as a separate and distinct portion of medical education, be abandoned, and that the internship and residency years be combined into a single period of graduate medical education called a residency and planned as a unified whole.[8]

These recommendations were put into effect during the decade after publication of the commission's report.

The approval of internships became a particularly sticky political issue because, although there were far too few of them to meet the demand, every hospital of any size wanted the services of interns in carrying out routine procedures. Early in the period under consideration there was a fairly good balance of United States graduates and approved internships, but as hospitals offered internships in increasing numbers, whether or not they were prepared to provide suitable educational opportunities, unfilled positions increased. While some were occupied by graduates of foreign schools, many remained vacant. By 1970, 15,354 approved internships were listed by the AMA, only 75 percent of which were filled. The appropriate position for the AMA to have taken would have been to confine approval to a number approximately equal to the number of graduates and ignore those that provided inadequate clinical opportunities, poor supervision, and poorly organized educational programs—but it was not politically expedient to do so.

Neither was the AMA very supportive of the medical schools in other respects during the post–World War II era. Fearful of the intrusion of the federal government in any aspect of medicine, it failed to support federal appropriations for operating funds, and endorsed with little enthusiasm appropriations for the construction of facilities. In summary, as it became more concerned with protecting the economic interests of practicing physicians it became less progressive in its concern for education.

THE SPECIALTY SOCIETIES

Another category of organizations that had some impact on the educational process was composed of the specialty societies —the American College of Surgeons, the American College of Physicians, the Academy of Pediatrics, the Academy of General Practice (later the Academy of Family Practice), and many others. While they were seldom concerned with predoctoral training, they played a significant role in determining the standards of residency training for specialization and providing opportunities for the continuing education of their members. At their national and regional meetings the specialty societies offered instruction in the form of lectures and demonstrations in which the scientific basis for, as well as application of, advances in knowledge were presented in a manner that was stimulating as well as instructive. They also took the leadership in providing opportunities for self-evaluation. As participation in these programs was voluntary, they reached those who had the greatest desire to learn and left unexposed many of those that needed it most. An exception to this generalization was the Academy of General Practice, which required a certain amount of participation in courses or educationally oriented meetings for continued membership. These organizations served a useful purpose in filling a vacuum in a phase of medical education that was largely neglected by the medical schools.

The elite societies with restricted memberships, such as the Association of American Physicians, the American Surgical Association, the American Pediatric Society, and the Society for Clinical Investigation, tended to be research oriented. Although composed of influential members of the medical academic fraternity, education was seldom mentioned in their transactions except in presidential addresses. The impact of these societies was probably greater than appeared on the surface, however, because conversations on the boardwalk and in the bars at Atlantic City during their annual meetings often determined the fate of curricular innovations, and the recruitment, as well as promotion, of younger and less-privileged faculty members.

FOUNDATIONS

The foundations, like the national professional organizations, while not engaged directly in medical education, were in a position to be of enormous influence. During the pre-World War II era they supported most of the research and contributed substantially to the remarkable development of many medical schools.

The most significant contributions during the period 1900 to 1930 were made by the foundations established by John D. Rockefeller. The three forerunners of the Rockefeller Foundation were the Rockefeller Institute for Medical Research (1901), the Rockefeller Sanitary Commission (1909), and the General Education Board (1903).

The Rockefeller Institute was dedicated to research and played no direct role in education. It was, however, an important source of scientifically trained personnel who filled several of the most prestigious chairs in the basic sciences and clinical medicine in the developing medical schools prior to World War II. In 1954 it became the Rockefeller University, an institution devoted to biomedical research and education at the graduate and postdoctoral levels.

The Sanitary Commission, founded for the purpose of eradicating hookworm infestation in the South, and its successor, the International Health Commission, played similar indirect roles in the development of education in public health.

The impact of the General Education Board on medical education was direct and extensive. After completing his survey, Abraham Flexner joined the Rockefeller staff: his mission was to establish full-time clinical departments in selected medical schools in the United States. This meant that for the first time clinical departments were to be under the administrative control of physicians or surgeons who would give all their time to teaching, research, and care of patients in teaching hospitals. If they saw private patients the fees received would go to the university. The first grant of this type was to the Johns Hopkins University in 1913; similar grants were made over the next decade to Yale, the University of Chicago, and Washington University. In 1923 the board provided funds for the centralization of the facilities of the State University of Iowa, and subsequently to other state universities and to black medical colleges.

The General Education Board was gradually phased out as its functions were taken over by the Rockefeller Foundation, founded in 1909

> . . . to promote the well-being and to advance the civilization of the peoples of the United States and its territories and possessions and of foreign lands in the acquisition of knowledge, in the prevention and relief of suffering, and in the promotion of any and all the elements of human progress.

Interest in the advancement of medical education was continued in the foundation's Division of Medical Sciences under the leadership of Richard M. Pearce, Alan Gregg, and Robert Morison.

For about twenty years, beginning in the 1930s, the Division of Medical Sciences devoted much of its attention to psychiatry, which at that time was isolated from other branches of medicine. Teaching and research in that field were of a low order, and were in fact virtually neglected in the curricula of most medical schools. Over the next several years departments of psychiatry were initiated or substantially aided at Harvard, the University of Chicago, McGill, Washington University, the University of Michigan, Tulane, Yale, and Johns Hopkins, and later at Columbia and the University of Colorado. This series of grants provides an excellent example of the way seeds are sown and pumps primed in educational circles. By the 1950s psychiatry had become a major clinical department, on a level with medicine and surgery, at most American medical schools.

Behind the scenes, Alan Gregg was a powerful influence in medical education during this period. His advice was sought about the establishment and reorganization of schools and the appointment of administrative officers and senior faculty members. His concern for quality in education and research kept the establishment on an even keel.

Programs supported by the Rockefeller Foundation for the study and control of infectious diseases led to an interest in the training of public health personnel. Prior to 1918 public health was unknown as a profession and there was no formal academic training in the discipline. To overcome this deficiency, in 1922 the foundation provided funds to establish the School of Hygiene and Public Health at Johns Hopkins and, over the next thirty years, twenty-one other schools of public health in the United States and abroad. Without doubt this program not only elevated the standards of public health service but promoted instruction in preventive medicine in medical schools by providing faculty members trained in that discipline. Whether the establishment of independent schools of public health was a good move from the standpoint of university organization is debatable. There was poor communication between the schools of public health and the medical schools, even when they were located on the same street, and many believe that more progress would have been made if the two faculties had been combined.

Another foundation established "to do something for the welfare of mankind" was the Commonwealth Fund, organized in 1918 and endowed by a series of gifts from Mrs. Stephen V. Harkness, her son, Edward S. Harkness, and his wife, Mary S. Harkness. Although not confined by charter or limited in its interests to medicine, the fund's major activity was in the health field, and during the first forty years of its existence it gave generous support to projects in medical research. As public concern with medical research grew rapidly, and as vast sums were made available by the federal government, the fund withdrew from extensive support for that purpose.

The Commonwealth Fund recognized from the beginning that medical education underlies all activities in the health field, and gave support to its improvement and expansion in a number of ingenious ways. In the postwar period most of its appropriations were in the field of medical education: it helped establish new schools; it encouraged the integration of the basic sciences with clinical instruction, and the medical school with other divisions of the university; it supported the development of the behavioral sciences and the teaching of comprehensive medicine; it encouraged research in medical education and the processes of learning; and it provided fellowships for advanced study by faculty members. Although it did not usually contribute funds for construction, the fund was broad enough in its views to recognize that on occasion lack of space may be the one factor that is holding back the development of an educational program, or that the morale of a student body and the atmosphere of an institution will be improved by the provision of decent living quarters.*

This may be as good a place as any to mention the importance of awarding unrestricted funds, an area in which the Commonwealth Fund set the example. In 1955 and 1956 it invaded its capital to make grants totaling $13,340,000 to nineteen private, nonsectarian, university-affiliated medical schools. A few schools placed the funds in permanent endowment; some used principal and interest over a period of years; many added faculty members or increased salaries; and some set up pilot experiments in education. The uses to which the funds were put were so varied that, in the group of schools as a whole, virtually every essential aspect of medical education was aided. The response of the schools to this type of giving, in contrast to the traditional project grants, was so

---

* I am personally indebted to the Commonwealth Fund for the assistance it provided in developing the physical plant of the Yale School of Medicine during the fifteen years I served as its dean. Grants for construction of the Edward S. Harkness Memorial Hall (a student dormitory), the Mary S. Harkness Auditorium, and the Laboratory of Clinical Investigation contributed immeasurably to improving morale and enhancing the educational and research programs.

enthusiastic that other foundations were inspired to take a similar course. In 1955 the Ford Foundation distributed $90 million in unrestricted funds directly to privately endowed medical schools, and another $10 million through the National Fund for Medical Education. Similar action was taken by the Josiah Macy, Jr. Foundation, the W. K. Mellon Foundation, and others.

The Macy Foundation, operating on a smaller scale than those mentioned previously, supported medical education consistently from the time of its founding in 1930. During the first thirty years it financed research in a wide variety of disciplines and on a number of disorders, particularly in the fields of growth and development, aging, and psychosomatic medicine. Like other private foundations, during the postwar period it gradually transferred its interest to education as federal funds for research became more plentiful. The foundation's sponsorship of well-organized invitational conferences, first on scientific topics and later on medical education, and the published reports of their deliberations, were among its most significant contributions. Other major interests were the development of teaching programs in the history of medicine and, in the late 1960s, the recruitment of students from disadvantaged minority groups for the study of medicine and the health-related professions.

The John and Mary R. Markle Foundation, founded in 1927, devoted its resources during the first twenty years to support of research. In 1946 John M. Russell became executive director of the foundation and conceived the Markle Scholar Program. Each medical school in the United States and Canada was invited to nominate a young man who had completed his training and was on the first rung of the academic ladder. On a regional basis, groups of candidates were assembled for weekends at resort hotels where they mingled with blue-ribbon panels of university presidents, business executives, and other notables, who made the final selection. It was assumed that endorsement by their parent institutions was sufficient evidence of the candidates' intelligence and scientific competence, so those chosen made the grade on the basis of their personalities. When Mr. Russell set up the program he prophesied that it would be considered successful if half the scholars attained leadership status in medical education or made important scientific contributions. Actually the results were much better, and to have been a Markle Scholar was recognized as a major distinction.

The scholarship award was for a period of five years, and at first amounted to $5,000 a year. In those early postwar days that amount was sufficient to cover the salary of an instructor and still leave funds available for support of his research and travel to a meeting or two. As salary levels increased, however, the stipends covered only a half or a quarter of an instructor's or assistant professor's salary, and to the scholar and his institution the financial reward became far less significant than the honor. The program was terminated in the late 1960s.

The National Fund for Medical Education (NFME) was organized in 1949, under the sponsorship of a group of university presidents and with the strong support of the AMA, AAMC, and "big business," for the purpose of seeking new sources of financial support for the medical schools. Five years later it was granted a federal charter by the Congress. During its first decade the NFME's leadership consisted of the heads of national industrial corporations, banks, airlines, utilities, and insurance companies, and it showed promise of becoming a major factor in the financing of medical education. The AMA made substantial annual contributions, and the Ford Foundation provided matching funds to encourage donations. As federal support for the operation of medical schools increased, however, the involvement of industry diminished. Initially the NFME distributed its income to all medical schools without restriction as to its use; later it made grants to encourage new methods of instruction and to improve efficiency of operation.

Many other foundations whose interests were not confined to medicine, such as the Kellogg Foundation, the Hartford Foundation, and the Kresge Foundation, also made important contributions to medical education and research during this period. Over the decade of the 1960s, foundation grants for health amounted to approximately $1 billion, $200 million of which went to medical education.[9]

As federal support became more substantial in the 1950s and 1960s, although foundation grants represented a small proportion of the medical schools' budgets they continued to be important because they supported programs and construction for which federal funds could not be obtained. Looking back over the entire fifty-year period it is difficult to identify any significant development in medical education in which a foundation grant did not play an important role.

NOTES

1. See: R. Shaplen, J. G. Harrar, and A. B. Tourtellot, *Toward the Well-Being of Mankind: Fifty Years of the Rockefeller Foundation* (New York: Doubleday, 1964); *The Commonwealth Fund: Historical Sketch, 1918–1962* (New York: The Commonwealth Fund, 1963); *The Josiah Macy, Jr. Foundation, 1930–1955* (New York: Josiah Macy, Jr. Foundation, 1955); M. Fishbein, *A History of the American Medical Association, 1847–1947* (Philadelphia: Saunders, 1947); J. H. Means, *The Association of American Physicians: Its First Seventy-Five Years* (New York: McGraw-Hill, 1961); and D. F. Smiley, "History of the Association of American Medical Colleges, 1876–1956," *Journal of Medical Education* 32 (1957): 520.

2. L. T. Coggeshall, *Planning for Medical Progress through Education* (Washington: Association of American Medical Colleges, 1965).

3. Commission on Medical Education, *Final Report of the Commission on Medical Education* (New York: Commission on Medical Education, 1932).

4. J. E. Dietrich and R. C. Berson, *Medical Schools in the United States at Mid-Century* (New York: McGraw-Hill, 1953).

5. American Psychiatric Association, *Psychiatry and Medical Education: 1951 Conference* (Washington: American Psychiatric Association, 1952); and *The Psychiatrist, His Training and Development: 1952 Conference* (Washington: American Psychiatric Association, 1953).

6. "The Teaching of Physiology, Biochemistry and Pharmacology" (1953); "The Teaching of Pathology, Microbiology, Immunology, and Genetics" (1954); "The Teaching of Anatomy and Anthropology" (1955); "The Appraisal of Applicants to Medical Schools" (1956); "The Ecology of the Medical Student" (1957);

"The First Institute on Clinical Teaching" (1958); "Medical Education and Medical Care" (1960); "Research and Medical Education" (1961); "Medical Education and Practice: Relationships and Responsibilities" (1962); "The First Institute on Medical School Administration" (1963); "The Second Administrative Institute: Medical School-Teaching Hospital Relations" (1964); "The Medical Center and the University" (1965); "Manpower for the World's Health" (1966); and "Family Planning and Medical Education" (1969).

7. H. G. Weiskotten et al., *Medical Education in the United States, 1934–1939* (Chicago: American Medical Association, 1940).

8. Citizens Commission on Graduate Medical Education, *The Graduate Education of Physicians: Report of the Citizens Commission on Graduate Medical Education* (Chicago: American Medical Association, 1966).

9. W. T. Swartz, "Foundations in the Changing World of Medical Education," *Foundation News* 13 (1972): 15.

XII. New Schools

IN 1920, eighty-six medical schools were in operation in the United States. Seventy-five offered the full four-year course and awarded the M.D. degree: * the remainder limited instruction to the first two, or preclinical, years and their students transferred to other schools for clinical instruction. Seventy-nine of the schools required two or more years of college work for admission; sixty-six were component units of universities; seventy-seven were regular or nonsectarian; five homeopathic; one eclectic; and three were classified as "nondescript affairs." Despite the improvement in the quality of most of the schools that had occurred over the previous decade there were still sixteen that did not meet even the minimal standards for full approval.[1]

It is interesting to note that forty years later, in 1960, there were still only eighty-six schools in operation. During the intervening years sixteen had closed their doors and been replaced by more viable institutions, and several of the two-year schools had expanded their clinical facilities and were offering the full four-year course.

One of the controversies that waxed and waned concerned the advisability of continuing in operation or of opening new two-year schools of the basic medical sciences. In their favor was the fact that there was always some attrition during the first two years, and that most four-year schools were prepared to accept a few transfers. As the division between preclinical and clinical studies became less distinct, however, and as more clinical work was introduced in the first two years, the status of the basic medical science schools was lowered. Nevertheless, the pressure to produce more doctors prompted some leaders

* Eleven required a fifth or internship year before award of the degree.

114

to advocate opening more of them. Only three additional schools of basic medical sciences were opened during that fifty-year period,* and in 1970 only six remained.†

Although seven medical schools were founded over the period 1920–1950,‡ conditions did not favor such expansion and at first there was an inclination to devote available resources to upgrading existing schools. Then came the economic depression and the war. With the end of the war and the return to prosperity in the 1950s the establishment of new schools became feasible; six new schools were opened during that decade.§

Applications for admission soared with the return of war veterans, but only half of those who applied could be admitted. Furthermore, opportunities for a medical education were not evenly distributed. In the nation as a whole, the ratio of students admitted in 1950 was 4.8 per 100,000 population; the ratios in individual states varied from 1.7 to 8.9. This was an embarrassing situation at a time when state universities were expanding rapidly, state and community colleges were being founded in large numbers, and the belief was widespread that higher education in any field should be available to all who wanted it.

Pressure to open new schools was also coming from other directions. Physicians educated in the pre-Flexnerian era, when medical graduates were in plentiful supply, were reaching the age of retirement, and communities, particularly in rural areas, that had always had a doctor found themselves

* Brown University (1963); University of Hawaii (1965); and Rutgers University (1966).

† Brown University; Dartmouth College; University of Hawaii; University of North Dakota; Rutgers University; and University of South Dakota.

‡ University of Rochester (1920); University of Chicago (1927); Duke University (1930); Louisiana State University (1931); University of Texas–Southwestern (1943); University of Washington (1945); and University of Puerto Rico (1949).

§ University of California at Los Angeles (1951); University of Miami (1952); University of Kentucky (1954); Albert Einstein College of Medicine (1955); University of Florida (1956); and New Jersey College of Medicine (1956).

without one. Underproduction in American schools was balanced to some extent by the emigration to European universities of American students who could not gain admission at home, and by the immigration of foreign physicians. The latter were welcomed by communities that needed medical services, but not by the families of students who had been denied admission to American medical schools.

Contrary to popular opinion, the establishment of new schools was not opposed by the medical profession. At the local level, state and county medical societies were often the strongest forces in mobilizing pressure on state legislatures to establish schools in state-supported universities and to appropriate funds for their construction. The AAMC, AMA, foundations, and deans of medical schools encouraged local interest by participation in surveys and by publication of well-documented reports that served as a basis for positive action. These reports, not all of which are recorded in the indexed medical literature, are valuable sources of information on the educational, social, economic, and demographic conditions that favored the establishment of new schools in particular localities.[2]

The economic advantages of having a medical center with its thousands of faculty, students, employees, and patients located in a small city were obvious, and chambers of commerce, representing business interests, often played major roles in promotion.*

By the late 1950s it became apparent that uncoordinated efforts to increase the production of physicians would not

---

* In the course of a study leading to the establishment of a state-supported medical school in Florida, I visited six cities. As a means of introduction I had been in contact with the presidents of the local medical societies. When I arrived, however, I was met and escorted by representatives of the chambers of commerce and city officials. My recommendation was that the school be located at the University of Florida in Gainesville. It was accepted by the state legislature, but, as a compromise, a rider to the bill provided for an operating subsidy of $3,000 per student for the *first* school opened. The University of Miami admitted its first class in outbuildings of the local veterans hospital six months later and obtained the subsidy. The University of Florida proceeded more deliberately and opened its medical center six years later.

satisfy the demand. The physician:population ratio had remained fairly constant over the previous fifty years, and some argued that it was adequate. Many infectious diseases had been brought under control by immunization, improved sanitation, and the introduction of antibiotics. Transportation and communication had improved, so that people who had previously depended on the village doctor and his horse and buggy could now be reached in a shorter time by a doctor from the county seat several miles away. On the other hand, there were more old people who required continuing care, and more diseases that were susceptible to treatment. The lay press as well as health authorities were beginning to show concern.[3]

It was realized that estimates of physician requirements based on demand alone, without consideration of need, were not reliable. Demand was interpreted as the amount of medical service people ask for spontaneously and can afford to pay for; need was defined as the amount of medical service, preventive and curative, necessary to provide optimal care for all the people. While few reliable studies of need had been made, isolated experiences indicated that when service was made available demand increased and more nearly approached need. The best that could be done was to base estimates of future requirements on maintenance of the current physician:population ratio.[4]

National commissions that produce voluminous reports are often ineffectual, but occasionally one that is organized at an opportune moment has great impact. The Surgeon General's Consultant Group on Medical Education was one such commission appointed at the right time. Its report, *Physicians for a Growing America*,[5] published in 1959, was influential in mobilizing public opinion and stirring the Congress into action. The ratio at that time was 133 M.D.'s and eight D.O.'s per 100,000 population, and the report concluded that if this ratio was to be maintained the number of graduates of medical and osteopathic schools annually would have to be increased from the present 7,400 to 11,000 by 1975. This would require the admission of 12,000 students a year by the fall of 1971.

In retrospect, there were at least two flaws in this estimate. It assumed that the United States would continue indefinitely to be dependent on the importation of foreign-trained physicians. (We should in fact have been exporting physicians to the developing countries instead of depriving them of their limited supply.) Furthermore, the population failed to increase during the next decade at the rate predicted, due, in part at least, to public acceptance of the concept of family planning.

The turning point was passage of the Health Professions Educational Assistance Act of 1963: one section provided matching funds for construction of facilities to establish new schools and expand existing ones. New schools were eligible to receive federal grants equal to two-thirds of the cost of construction and the basic equipment for essential teaching facilities, including teaching hospitals; existing schools could apply for one-half the cost. The appropriations were far from sufficient to meet the demand, and in very few instances were the allocations of federal funds actually in the proportion permitted by law.

In awarding these grants the custom of appointing advisory councils to review proposals, examine plans, and visit the applicant institutions followed the pattern that had proved so successful in the funding of research projects by the National Institutes of Health. High standards of efficiency in allocation of space and relationship of functions were required, and architectural plans that did not meet the minimal requirements for net to gross space ratios were returned promptly for redesign. (Net space was that within the walls of functional areas such as laboratories, classrooms, and offices; gross space was the interior of the entire building, including corridors, elevators, toilets, etc., for common use.) Although many handsome medical school buildings were erected during the 1960s, their esthetic qualities were a tribute to the architects' ingenuity and local contributions, rather than to extravagant use of federal funds.

During the decade 1960 through 1969, entering classes matriculated at fifteen new medical schools,* bringing the total number of schools in operation during the academic year 1969–70 to 101. Twelve others were under development.[6]

The cost of constructing and operating medical schools had become so prohibitive that few privately endowed universities had the resources or the courage to enter this field of education: only four of the twenty-one schools opened in the 1950s and 1960s were sponsored privately. Even some of those classified as private, first in Pennsylvania, Ohio, and Florida, and later in other states, received state subsidies for operation.

Increased dependence on tax funds for support did not, fortunately, adversely affect the freedom of the schools to reorganize their administrations or adopt new curricula or methods of instruction. In contrast to the situation in many other countries, where support was derived entirely from national governments, central control of medical education was avoided. The freedom to innovate that characterized the American system can be attributed to the fact that support was obtained from a diversity of governmental units, and even state-supported institutions could acquire funds for new approaches from foundations and other private sources.

The opening of new schools was only one factor that led to the increased enrollment and production of physicians. In the 1960s federal funds for unrestricted use were made available on a capitation basis to schools that increased the size of their entering classes by 5 percent.

The effects of federal subsidies for construction of educational facilities and for operation soon became apparent. In

---

* University of New Mexico (1960); Brown University (1963); Medical College of Ohio at Toledo (1964); Michigan State University (1966); Rutgers University (1966); Louisiana State University at Shreveport (1966); University of Arizona (1967); Pennsylvania State University (1967); University of Hawaii (1967); University of Texas at San Antonio (1968); Mount Sinai School of Medicine (1968); University of California at Davis (1968); University of California at San Diego (1968); University of Connecticut (1968); and University of Texas at Houston (1969). (The dates noted are years of organization rather than the years when the first classes were matriculated.)

1959–60, 8,173 students were enrolled in entering medical school classes, and 7,081 were graduated; by 1969–70, entering students numbered 10,401, and 8,367 graduated. The requirements established by the Surgeon General's Consultant Group in 1959 were exceeded in the following year, and, as all new schools were operated during the first few years at less than capacity, the potential rate of production was considerably higher.

Thus, over the fifty-year period, 1920–1970, the number of physicians graduated annually had increased by a multiple of 2.74 (3,047 to 8,367), while the population of the country had grown by a multiple of 2. Graduating classes of at least 14,000 in 1980, 69 percent above the 1970 level, appeared to be assured. After a long era of dependence on the importation of physicians educated in other countries, there was at last a promise of self-sufficiency.

NOTES

1. A. D. Bevan, "Report of the Council on Medical Education," *Journal of the American Medical Association* 74 (1920): 1243.

2. The following are examples; there are many others: J. F. Volker, *The Arizona Medical School Study* (Tucson: University of Arizona Press, 1962); V. W. Lippard, *Education for the Health Services of the State of Florida* (Tallahassee: Florida State Board of Education and State Board of Control, 1949); J. N. Boone and M. S. Woods, *Medical Education for Tennessee* (Nashville: Tennessee Higher Education Commission, 1971); New York State Committee on Medical Education, *Education for the Health Professions* (Albany: New York State Education Department, 1963); and V. W. Lippard, W. R. Berryhill, and J. C. Hinsey, *Medical Education in South Carolina* (Columbia: Commission on Higher Education, 1967).

3. "Shortage of Doctors?" *U.S. News and World Report* 44, no. 19 (May 9, 1958).

4. The 54th Congress on Medical Education and Licensure, held in Chicago in February 1958, was devoted to consideration of the problem of the future production of physicians. A series of papers and workshop reports summarizing the prevailing attitudes and opinions was published in the *Journal of the American Medical Association* 167 (1958): 21-57.

5. The Surgeon General's Consultant Group on Medical Education, *Physicians for a Growing America* (Washington: U.S. Government Printing Office, Public Health Service Publication No. 709, 1959).

6. For a detailed account of the problems involved in starting a new medical school at this time, see: V. W. Lippard and E. Purcell, eds., *Case Histories of Ten New Medical Schools* (New York: Josiah Macy, Jr. Foundation, 1972).

Epilogue

TWENTY years ago I would have felt comfortable in predicting the future of medical education over the next two decades. Medical science was progressing at a rapid pace, and carefully selected students were taking good advantage of the opportunities to become scientifically oriented physicians. Medical school catalogs stated that the primary purpose of the standard four-year curriculum was to provide the student with a sound background in biological sciences and clinical medicine that would prepare him to adapt to the continued advances in medical science that could be anticipated. Medical faculties were becoming increasingly concerned with expanding their research programs, as what appeared to be inexhaustible support was becoming available.

Today everything is changing and the future is far less predictable. Even the student body is becoming more heterogeneous as admissions policies are becoming more relaxed in order to accommodate students with a wider range of preparation as well as social and ethnic backgrounds.

The roles of various health professionals and the interrelationship of these roles are also changing. One result of this trend may be that the discrete organization of the medical faculty will cease to exist and be absorbed into a much broader faculty concerned with the education of health workers with a spectrum of backgrounds and interests. The traditional departmental organization is threatened as the boundaries between the disciplines become less distinct and interdisciplinary instruction more common.

The core curriculum introduced during the past few years is resulting in diminished emphasis on the basic sciences, and in an effort to produce more physicians faster the medical course is being abbreviated. These changes are, in my estimation, misguided. Whether or not they will persist is uncertain. A system that produces physicians with a wider variety of levels of competence seems imminent.

The curricula of some new schools look very much like the programs for training physician's assistants. If the latter are to assume much of the responsibility for routine procedures requiring technical skills rather than judgment, and if physicians are to be engaged primarily in decision making, there is good reason to believe that the physician of the future should be educated in even greater depth scientifically than he has been in the past. Furthermore, it is difficult to conceive how he can be expected to keep up with advances in the biological sciences if he lacks a sound scientific foundation.

Serious mistakes of American medical education during the past several decades have included the overproduction of many types of specialists; the fragmentation of specialties; and the failure to produce primary physicians—general internists, pediatricians, and family physicians—in adequate numbers. Physicians prepared to accept responsibility for continuing care and health management are in short supply. As a national health program evolves, particularly if it is characterized by widespread utilization of health maintenance organizations, the demand for physicians of this type will increase and opportunities for specialized practice diminish. Hopefully, the production of specialists and their geographical distribution will be regulated.

When all the new schools that opened around 1970 are operating at full capacity, the demand for medical services should be satisfied without the importation of an appreciable number of those trained overseas. Residency training programs will be limited to hospitals affiliated with medical schools, and will be brought into balance with the number of American graduates.

The continuum of medical education, widely discussed but inadequately implemented, will become a reality. More students will enter medical school having taken courses in biochemistry and cell biology, for example, comparable to those offered first-year medical students. Formal education will not terminate with award of the M.D. degree or certification by a specialty board, and the practicing physician will be forced to keep up with advances by periodic reexamination for continued licensure.

The financial problems of our medical schools are likely to persist. The universities have never fully accepted medical education as their financial responsibility: medical schools have been tolerated as long as they paid their own way and did not disturb community relations. Federal support for educational purposes has been, and probably will continue to be, unreliable. The country may eventually realize that the education of health personnel, like the provision of medical care for all segments of the population, is a national responsibility. Complete federal support of medical schools is neither necessary nor desirable, but predictable basic support on a capitation basis is needed to provide the kind of foundation for programming that is so essential.

Most needed at this time is the development of a national system for the distribution of health services based on the concept of equal accessibility and availability for all citizens. If and when that is accomplished, a rational program for educating health manpower to meet the requirements of that system can be designed.[1]

NOTES

1. For more extensive predictions of the future of medical education, written at about the same time that this book was in preparation, see: J. B. Richmond, *Currents in American Medicine* (Cambridge: Harvard University Press, 1969); J. S. Millis, *A Rational Public Policy for Medical Education and Its Financing* (New York: National Fund for Medical Education, 1971); and W. G. Anlyan et al., *The Future of Medical Education* (Durham: Duke University Press, 1973).

Index